CW00822152

This Small Life

A Woman's Healing Journey

Barbara Hayes

Pottersfield Press

Copyright © Barbara Hayes 2002

All rights reserved. No part of this publication may be reproduced or transmitted in any form or by any means, electronic or mechanical, including photocopying, or by any information storage or retrieval system, without permission in writing from the publisher.

National Library of Canada Cataloguing in Publication Data
Hayes, Barbara
       This small life: a woman's healing journey

ISBN 1-895900-47-6

1. Hayes, Barbara 2. Psychosynthesis. 3. Arthritis—Patient—
Nova Scotia—Biography. 4. Antigonish (N.S.)—Biography. I. Title.

RC933.H39 2002   362.1 '96722'0092   C2002-900396-2

Pottersfield Press gratefully acknowledges the ongoing support of the Nova Scotia Department of Tourism and Culture, Cultural Affairs Division, as well as The Canada Council for the Arts. We acknowledge the financial support of the Government of Canada through the Book Publishing Industry Development Program for our publishing activities.

Printed in Canada

Pottersfield Press
83 Leslie Road
East Lawrencetown
Nova Scotia, Canada, B2Z 1P8
Website: www.pottersfieldpress.com

To order, telephone toll free 1-800-NIMBUS9 (1-800-646-2879)

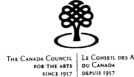
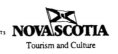
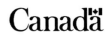

I am so small I can barely be seen.
How can this great love
be inside me?
Look at your eyes. They are small,
But they see enormous things.

Rumi

This book is dedicated to the memory of my mother and my sister Irene, and to my children, Jesse, Seamus, and Sidonie.

This Small Life : A Woman's Healing Journey

Table of Contents

Preface: The Importance of Telling Our Stories

Telling stories is a very human way of sharing and connecting with one another. As long as there have been people, there have been stories and storytellers. Long ago, humans gathered together around their fires and regaled one another with stories of trial, challenge, triumph, loss, love, daring, beauty, and all things sacred. Telling stories was a way of passing on wisdom, knowledge, and traditions, a way of making sense of events, of rendering them repeatable, memorable, significant. Indeed, we all remain in the thrall of stories, both our own and others'. And for good reason. When we tell our own stories, or listen to the personal stories of others, we are participating in meaning-making events. By recounting our experience of the events of our lives, we make sense of what has happened to us; we find the threads that weave the fabric of who we are together. Chance becomes plan; as we begin to see and understand the patterns within which we live, we begin to be able to live more consequently, to choose more knowingly, to take wiser rather than more foolish risks. But to discover all of this, we must have the opportunity to tell our stories, to listen and to be listened to.

As Rachel Naomi Remen says in her collection of life-changing tales, *Stories That Heal:*

So many of us do not know our own story. A story about who we are, not what we have done. About what we have faced to build what we have built, what we have drawn upon and risked to do it, what we have felt, thought, feared and discovered throughout the events of our lives: the real story that belongs to us alone.

This Small Life is one such story; it is my story about questing, about searching for the ultimate meaning and force in life, my life. It tells of a journey from loneliness and isolation from the self, the heart of sadness, to connection, self-discovery and love, the heart of light. And while this story is a personal journey, it contains many features that others will recognize: here are many stopping places and questions; there are stumbling blocks, confusions; here disaster opens onto life-changing realizations and new pathways for inquiry and action, new understandings and routes to becoming more truly human. The themes of my story are not uncommon then; they share much with countless other stories that have been written or told throughout time. This story asks many of the same questions that have been asked repeatedly before: Who am I? What is life about? Why is there such suffering and what is its meaning? How can I find meaning, peace, serenity, and come to joy and self-acceptance? In seeking my own answers to these questions, I turned to others' writings, others' life stories, others' wisdom, much of which counseled me to look deep within myself for the sources of my pain, and my healing, without, however, leaving me entirely on my own. My debts to others then are enormous; without the physical, psychic, and spiritual support of numerous friends, family members, and inspirational and talented healthcare workers, this journey would not have been possible. I am especially grateful to friends, fellow students in Psychosynthesis, and my teachers, especially Olga Denisko. I am also grateful to my close women friends who encouraged me to write, to Vangie Babin, who did the first typing of this manuscript, to Dorothy Thompson, who did the corrections, to my clients who have taught me so much, and to all those friends and healthcare workers in Massachusetts and Canada who supported and sustained me on this journey. My everlasting thanks to Karin Cope, who helped me to shape the fragments of my story into a coherent whole. And last, but far from least, I owe a debt of gratitude to my partner Chris, who always encouraged me to continue. Certain books and phrases have also traveled alongside me, important companions on my life's journey; they are noted as they are mentioned in the text.

If a life is conceived as a journey, then its telling may be understood as the drawing of a map, useful both to the one journeying as well as for those who follow. It is my hope that this little book, which chronicles some of my own psychical, physical, and spiritual struggles, may also serve others in valuing and making a record of their own life journeys, and help to persuade them to add their own tales, signs, and guideposts to the storehouse of shared human wisdom and experience.

INTRODUCTION: Finding Our True Nature

We are all self-actualizing beings! In simple terms, our purpose in life is to uncover our potential, our gifts, and share them with the world. That is what Abraham Maslow wrote in his influential book, *Toward a Psychology of Being*. We are also here in this lifetime to work toward finding our true nature, the divine within us. This quest and legacy has come down to us through the ages in many forms and guises, all of which suggest that '*We are much more than we seem.*' We have a dimension to our nature that is more than our everyday survival-selves. This dimension has been described as a search for deeper purpose and meaning; it is in fact a search for spiritual life. Maslow contended that the spiritual life was part of our human essence, that it was a defining characteristic of human nature. The search for this aspect of our nature is the journey of self-actualization, of greater spiritual knowledge and awareness. Some of us become aware of this aspect of ourselves at an early age while many more come to it later in life. For some of us, it takes an illness or near death experience to bring into focus the existence of an 'other reality.'

Once the first glimmer of such a spiritual awakening or awareness is seen, everything one has known previously can be thrown into question. In the late 1960s, I had what I would now

describe as a mystical experience through the use of an hallucinogenic drug. It was part of *"the scene"* at the time, of course, but the
experience changed my view of the world from that moment on. At
the time I was living with a group of people who were experimenting with different ways of living and being. Trying out drugs was
part of that process, but far from its end.

I had what would be described by Maslow as a peak or
mystical experience, in which I felt intimately a part of the universe. I saw my natural surroundings—trees, rocks, clouds, plants,
animals—all radiating an energy that was interconnected. Everything was alive and breathing, and I was part of it: *"I was at one
with the universe."* It was a startling, wonderful, and in some
ways terrifying experience. It changed my life! It put into question
the nature of reality. Which was the true reality: my everyday self,
or the self that experienced that incredible sensation of being a part
of everything? I knew that I was a being of energy. I knew that
everything in the universe was made from this same energy. But to
see this energy radiating from everything I looked at and touched
was both awesome and scary. Rocks were breathing, trees were
dancing; it was so wonderful that it was divine. Like Walt
Whitman, I "sang the body electric"; I was in the world and it was
in me. Like Whitman, I would sing,

> *Mine is no callous shell,*
> *I have instant conductors all over me whether I pass or*
> *stop,*
> *They seize every object and lead it harmlessly through me.*
> *I merely stir, press, feel with my fingers, and am happy'.*
> ("Song of Myself," lines 614-17)

I went on to have several experiences of this nature with
drugs, which I believe awoke in me a longing that became part of
my life. This longing was the quest for my true nature, the space of
the spiritual, the divine, within me.

As this book will relate, over the subsequent twenty-five
years, I kept straying from and re-connecting with the spiritual part
of my existence. But it was not until the onset of a chronic

debilitating illness in 1989-90 that a new way of being and living emerged. This new way of being continues to unfold in my life. I still suffer from the disease which manifested itself more than a decade ago; I have not cured myself or been cured by a natural holistic therapy, nor have I been brought into remission by some spiritual realization or transcendence. There are, I am sure, many reasons why this has not happened. As I have struggled with my illness, I *have* found healing, if not the eradication of what ails my body. I have moved nearer to acceptance of what is, rather than holding on to an impossible and stubborn idealization of a prior, imagined state of health. As Rilke so wisely asked in his *Letters to a Young Poet,*

> *Why do you want to shut out of your life any agitation, any pain, any melancholy since you really do not know what these states are working upon you?*

I am still just beginning to realize, after more than a decade, what these states—this illness with all of its accompanying changes, losses, terrors and joys— are working on me. I am just beginning to realize what life is teaching me through this process of trial and discovery. The writing of this small book has been a part of that process of trial and discovery, the journey of healing in which I discover what my true strengths and resources are, and how I might best make use of them. Reflecting upon one's life is a part of a healing process: you may revisit old wounds, old sorrows, old angers with compassion and understanding; they become not simply evils to be uprooted or overcome, but instruments in your awakening. *This Small Life* is, then, the story of my quest for greater self-awareness, greater aliveness, greater compassion for myself and others. In short, it is a story of healing and self-actualization.

Like many, I wanted to be healed, but I confused healing with being cured, with ridding myself of the noxious illness that was plaguing me. But as I struggled with the things that my body could no longer do, I gained all sorts of insights. I realized that in my most, so-called, healthy, vibrant state, I had not been at peace with who I was. I was driven, angry, controlling. My self-loathing was mixed up in my efforts to eradicate violence and misogyny in the community where I lived. I went about trying to fix in the world what I had not fixed in myself; I tried to rid the world of an "old" way of life without imagining I must lay the groundwork for a new one on the scarred terrain where the old life had been. If the personal was political, the political was also personal, and there was no time for anything else, certainly no time for compassion for my own frailties or those of anyone else. There was a world to save, now! Here! The youthful passion I had for life had an element of neurosis, of compulsion within it; I could not find peace. It took my illness to bring about a more than transitory spiritual awakening, for the challenges my illness presented to my body opened the way for me to begin to work with my whole person, body, mind, feelings, *and* soul.

Over the course of the last decade, I have struggled with acceptance of my illness as part of my life, part of who I am. I continue, of course, to eat a healthy diet, to follow a health and exercise regime to keep my body as active as I can, but I have come to accept the fact that this challenging and painful arthritic condition may stay with me for the rest of my life. I also realize that I can live in peace with that knowledge. I know it will not or does not impede my growth, that it cannot constrain how I do the work I feel most called to do: to share this knowledge of the fullness of being with others.

My renewed sense of spiritual aliveness does not mean that I don't fall into old patterns, old angers and despairs; it does not mean that I have escaped once and for all the "dark night of soul." Still, in the course of my healing journey, a journey that has involved not only therapies of various sorts but also training as a therapist who is attuned to spiritual strivings as well as psychological needs, I have acquired some tools that help me to continue on my way. When I have self-doubts now, I am able to stop and ask myself: according to what exhausted standard am I striving? Can I accept being who I am, and know that is enough? I don't have to save the world, as I thought I had to in the past. Not only can I be human but that is who I am; it is my calling. Everything I do must start here. Being human means not only that I compassionately accept and embrace my own history and struggles, my own frailties and failings, but also that I nurture my strengths, my feelings of wonder. I allow my glories to shine, and the glory of the world through me.

This then is what I have to offer here to myself, to my readers, and to the people who come to consult me in my practice: the reminder of the wisdom of viewing human nature through a transformational rather than pathological lens. Our angers, self-hatreds, addictions, fears, weaknesses, illnesses and longings are all part of our human wealth and inheritance; these things shape our strivings. Suffering is common to us all; joy also is accessible to us all. What matters, in the search for greater wisdom and healing, is how we make use of our experiences of suffering and joy.

It is worth it perhaps, as we seek and strive, to remember that

Our deepest fear [may] not be that we are inadequate. Our deepest fear [may be] that we are powerful beyond measure. It is our light, not our darkness, that most frightens us. We ask ourselves, "Who am I to be brilliant, gorgeous, talented, fabulous?" Actually, who are you not to be? You are a child of God. Your playing small doesn't serve the world. There's nothing enlightened about shrinking so that other people won't feel insecure around you. We are all meant to shine as children do. We were born to make manifest the glory of God that is within us. It's not just in some of us, it's in everyone. And as we let our own light shine, we unconsciously give other people permission to do the same. As we're liberated from our own fear, our presence automatically liberates others. *

CHAPTER I
The Journey Begins

A Chaotic Childhood

All of us experience abandonment in some form; we cannot live every moment of our lives having all our needs met. Consequently, we have all experienced unfulfilled needs, and in our early developmental years these unmet needs represent abandonment. Even if these unmet needs are not, strictly speaking, life threatening, we carry the memory of them—the sensation of abandonment—with us into our adult lives; it haunts us, threatens us, informs our deepest emotions and actions. In time, if these feelings are not recognized and addressed, particularly if one's childhood was traumatic, and one also carries other wounds alongside the feelings of abandonment, those feelings and that history *can* threaten one's well-being, one's ability to be at peace with oneself, and to build sustaining relationships with others. A part of any healing journey then is not simply surviving such wounds when they first occur, but being able to recognize and name them when they recur, and learning to see, understand, and accept where they have come from: in short, to discover and to tell one's own story, one's own roots and history.

In my case, the characteristics of these early wounds were largely due to the chaotic nature of the emotional environment which was my home: an alcoholic father, a depressed and angry mother, both of them bound together, catastrophically, by the strict and repressive Roman Catholic culture of 1950's rural Ireland. Women were politically powerless; they were counseled and conditioned to obey their husbands and fathers—God's representative in the home. Sex was considered sinful for a woman even in marriage. My upbringing was thus sewn through with strong themes of misogyny and bodily self-hatred.

As I think about it now, it seems to me that I endured great loneliness and confusion. It was hard for a passionate and active girl to make sense of any of the roles or the life that might be left to her as a woman. The role that was exalted was the sainted Irish mother: self-sacrificing, patient, and forever caring for others' needs before her own. What I inherited from my own mother was a nagging feeling that selfishness was the greatest of sins, that to take time and space for oneself was selfish, to insist upon such a thing was sinful. In our Ireland, to develop one's self as a woman was a near impossibility. To be a self-determined adult and a woman was a contradiction in terms.

I was born the youngest of my parents' six children—three boys and three girls— in a small town on the edge of the bog of Allan in southern Ireland. By the time I was ten years old, my next older sister, Irene, had moved to England to find work, and my eldest sister, Lynn, had gone to Canada. Going to England or America for work was not uncommon then for young people who lived in rural Ireland; there was not much work, particularly for young women who were not yet married, where we lived. I think now that the scattering of her children must have been very hard on my mother.

My earliest memories are of summer, among them very vivid recollections of riding with my grandfather—*Hagga* as we called him— to the bog. He kept a horse and trap, and worked as a groom at the house of Anglo-Irish gentry in our town. The bog then was really quite a wonderful place: an incredible ecosystem of birds, plants, marshes and so many butterflies! I can still vividly recall the scents and sounds of driving along the road to the bog: the clip-clopping of the horse's feet, the smell of leather and horse sweat, the rhythmic motion of the horse trotting, the jingle of the harness. If I was lucky, I would be allowed to hold the reins.

My maternal grandfather was quiet and steady and very much in control. He brooked no argument from man or beast. When we drove into the bog, we had to traverse some very wet spots, and he would rail at the horse to keep her moving. He was stern but kindly, and I obeyed him without question. He had married a Protestant woman who had converted to Catholicism. I believe she obeyed him without question for the most part, although even in those days, women had ways of working around men to get what they wanted.

An outing to the bog was a very special event to me. When we drove there so that my grandfather could cut turf, I would be allowed to jump out of the trap and collect wild flowers and gorse as he stacked the turf to dry. In those days, turf was cut by hand with a slane. It had a great clean smell as it dried, and a fragrant smell when it was burned as fuel. Years later when I went back to Ireland and visited the bog with my cousin Danny, I was shocked by the devastation that machine cutting had caused; the bog was no longer the life-filled and beautiful place that I remembered.

My grandparents lived at the other end of town, and my grandmother would come to visit my mother at least once a week. Invariably, my grandmother arrived dressed in black and violet, and she always wore a hat with a huge hatpin that she would remove before she took her hat off. She was slender and erect, if not a particularly tall woman. My grandmother would often confer with my mother in whispered undertones, perhaps placating my mother, urging her to endure. Sometimes she would give my mother a small amount of money from her purse for Mother's personal use. Often my mother would ask me to walk part of the way home with my grandmother, and I remember that my grandmother often gave me some pennies or sweets from her pockets. I would have been about eight or nine years old at that time.

My grandfather sometimes came up to visit on Saturday

mornings if it was Fair day—meaning there would be a local farmers' fair in the town square. We lived in a house in the town square. I remember my mother buying a live turkey at Christmas, which she then killed and cleaned herself for our Christmas dinner. On Fair days, *Hagga* would come up to look at the horses and to talk to various farmers, then he came to our house for some refreshment. My mother often made him an egg flip: hot milk into which a beaten egg was poured, and if she had it, a good shot of whiskey and a little sugar. This drink would fortify *Hagga* and give him the energy he needed to make the walk back home in cold weather.

The town square was the scene of many events, from dances in the town hall to altars erected for the Corpus Christi Procession. These latter were my favorite events: the processions involved hundreds of flowers, which would then be pinned to white satin cloths to decorate the altars. The dances were also exciting because I could look out my bedroom window and see people arriving all dressed up, hear the bands playing, and the noise of the parties. But if the truth be told, times were rare when something so exciting happened.

The cinema was also in the town square, and occasionally, if she had a little extra cash, my mother would take me there. My mother loved musicals; I particularly remember seeing *The King and I*, *Carousel*, and *South Pacific* with her. She also often took me for walks at night after supper, and during the long summer evenings we might walk up Clonmullen Lane and through the fields outside of town. These were very precious times with my mother; they usually only happened when my father was away working. I loved my mother with great passion, and I savored these moments alone with her. They are very bright memories of times of great happiness in our lives.

Summer evenings were long in that part of Ireland. It would remain light till at least 10:15 p.m. There was time for jaunts on the bicycle or to roam the countryside. Occasionally in mid-summer, we might swim in the river with other children from the neighbourhood. Ireland has a very beautiful pastoral countryside, and in the 1950s, I remember that it was still very unspoiled. I was able to enjoy where I was, peacefully, as long as my father was away from home.

But when he returned from a job elsewhere, we all lived in fear, awaiting the inevitable binge of drinking and his angry and violent outbursts. Mother would warn us to be quiet and keep out of his way when he was drinking, but even quiet avoidance could not always help me. I had already learned to feel ashamed of my body thanks to the admonitions of the church, where it seemed one was always at risk of committing sins of impurity, having impure thoughts, and doing impure actions. Such an incessantly drilled sense of sinfulness, combined with my father's inappropriate touching of me and his violations of my privacy, confused and shamed me many times over. I did not tell any of these feelings or events to the priest in the confessional— which meant, of course, that I lived with an unrelieved sense of sinfulness: I was somehow bad beyond all redemption.

I think such feelings of general and irremediable wickedness were a common experience for many children in Ireland in those days, nurtured by a common cultural obsession with sins of the flesh: the confusion of sexuality with sin, the projection of this sinful sexuality onto children far too young to comprehend what was happening, the probing questions asked by priests, who seemed, themselves, fascinated by accounts of sins of impurity. The sense of guilt and shame, a conviction of one's own awfulness, seemed inevitable for those raised in such straightened and repressive Catholic communities. As a child, I would try to put the feelings of my own badness and shame from my mind when I went to church, as if these feelings were inadmissible there. What I could not see is that the church had its own large role in the inculcation of those feelings; they were not feelings at odds with the church so much as feelings implanted and encouraged by the church.

As a child, I was frightened by my father's anger, though I was not afraid that he would beat me; I was not afraid for myself, but I was frightened by the intensity of his emotions, the sheer size and ferocity of his rage. Of course, as a child observing such large adult emotions, I did not yet have the equipment to understand what was really going on, my father's great depression, loss of self-esteem, and despair. Sometimes huge fights would break out between my father and my mother. When they happened at night, I could not sleep and I sat in my nightdress at the top of the stairs, shivering and terrified. These were very bleak times.

The struggle to survive, accompanied by pervasive alcoholism, was a familiar enough condition for generations of families in Ireland. And in that environment, I, like so many others, set my course for survival, if little more. What supported my survival was the joy I found in the beautiful countryside, and my retreat into the world of my imagination. I read constantly, and from the ages of twelve to seventeen, I hungrily consumed the vast wealth of several centuries of English and Irish writers and poets. I particularly loved the Romantic poets, for they described for me the feelings I had of losing myself in the beauties of the countryside. Literature, I learned, provided a great escape; it became a space of joy, a habit of excursion, of flight, that has sustained and educated me throughout my life.

When I was not reading, I roamed the countryside, playing in ruins of castles and walking by rivers and ponds. I had a fascination with wild birds, with herons, swans, hawks, and eagles. My head was full of stories of Irish mythology: the legends of the Red Branch Knights and Warrior Queens, of saints and scholars, holy wells, banshees, and the little people. All of these places and creatures, both imaginary and real, helped me to split off from and tolerate the more painful and fearful aspects of my life.

During my last years in Ireland, when I was between the ages of twelve and fourteen, my father was away, working in England. My sister, Irene, who features prominently in my life story, had also moved to England, as had my three older siblings. Only the littlest ones, my brother and me, lived at home with our mother. During this time I remember that I struggled with loneliness and confusion, as perhaps many young adolescents do. I didn't know what would become of me.

When my father returned and my mother decided to leave him, the situation between them had deteriorated considerably. My father's violence and alcohol abuse had increased over the years, and as he aged, he became a very lost and beaten man, full of anger and pain. As was common enough, I suppose, he vented his anger, pain, and disappointment on his wife and children for years, until it became too dangerous for any of us to remain. My father's drinking had started early in his adult life, after he returned home from serving in the trenches during the First World War. He had been seventeen when he went away to war and survived its nightmares, and his experiences, about which little was ever said, changed him forever. Today we might classify my father's responses to the effects of the horror he had lived through as understandable expressions of Post-Traumatic Stress Syndrome. But in the time and place where he lived, there was little or no help for him or others like him, save the drowning he could give his history and emotions in the bottom of a bottle. Alcohol was what he turned to as a defense against feeling.

As a result of the last violent encounter between my parents, a battle which drove my mother out of her home to England with my brother and me, my mother, however briefly, asserted her right to freedom and selfhood. Hers was a socially dangerous decision, because a good Catholic wife does not leave her husband, no matter what, and while it saved her life (and ours) in one way perhaps, it destroyed it in another, for she carried immense guilt and self-reproach with her for the rest of her life. All of us too in our various ways have shouldered or struggled with this guilt and self-reproach as well. They have been, it seems, a part of our familial inheritance, an embedded piece of our histories among the elements that have shaped how our lives have unfolded.

The Hand of Fate

When I left Ireland at the age of fourteen, I was scared and unsure of myself, as I suppose many people are at such an age, particularly when they are so suddenly and violently uprooted. I was entering the unknown. It felt as if I were a matchstick and a giant hand had lifted me from the steady river stream where I drifted, and thrown me into a raging torrent, where I went rushing headlong, over the edge and into a falls. The next six years were spent trying desperately to keep afloat. From my perspective at the time, our move was disastrous. In retrospect, however, whether accident or fate, that move was a crucial part of my growth and development. Much of what was to follow unfolded from it.

The key players in this new scene of my adolescence were my mother and my sister, Irene. The connection between the three of us would continue for years, as we became the three sides of a triangle of intense and shared experiences, this long after I left home and we ceased to share any geographic proximity.

My mother, brother, and I settled in the south of England, in the glorious Devon countryside, in a delightful regency coastal town. Even so, I was scared. Terrified. I was afraid that our father would follow us and get us, harm us. Again, I was fortunate to be surrounded by great natural beauty; it helped me to endure the pain, anxiety, and loss of all the familiar things I had known: my home, my town, relatives, friends, and the countryside all around, those fields and familiar haunts that I felt were mine, and now no longer available to me. In this new country where we settled, I did not have a sense of belonging; I could not call it my own. Very different from the wild countryside of Ireland, nevertheless, the beauty in Devon was breathtaking. I was plunged into a life of solitude, where, once more, books and nature were my solace and closest companions.

At fourteen years of age, I was a healthy Irish girl with a strong accent. I attended the local grammar school, but I didn't fit in well. I was quiet, bookish and utterly self-conscious about my Irish accent. People often said that they could not understand me. I was keenly aware of my family's poverty, and I constantly felt out of place, like a fish out of water. My element was the wilds of Ireland, where I could roam the lush green countryside with my books. And in Ireland, I had loved my school. It was the one steady human center in my chaotic young life. There I was valued and affirmed. There I was somebody: an intelligent student who got good marks. There I found order and consistency and was introduced to literature and poetry, which transported me to other realms of knowledge, sensuality, and delight.

The first thing I found in the beautiful, conservative English town that was my new home was the old church library. Volunteers, mostly women in their seventies, ran it. Crammed with stacks of old books, the library was in a gorgeous old building badly in need of repair. Books ranged from the floor to the high vaulted ceiling; you had to climb a rickety ladder to reach the topmost volumes. The church library was a free library, and quite separate from the town library. There, I could be as anonymous as I wished. Very few people used this library, and most of those who did were well over seventy years of age. There were stacks of old books for sale there too, available for a pittance. I bought what I could and my constant reading resumed. I continued to read at least two books a week for the next several years, until the practice became a habit that has continued most of my life.

At school, in addition to my shame about our poverty and my "ignorant" Irish accent, I did not find a teacher to be a mentor. The school was not up to the standard of the convent school I had attended in Ireland. I remember that I was teased a good deal— mostly it was simple schoolgirl banter— but by then I was hypersensitive and almost afraid to speak. Terrified of further ridicule, I felt I could not reveal myself or my passion for music and literature, so I withdrew into solitude, and often felt desperately unhappy. Indeed, one of the few consistent bright spots in my schooldays was the hot-cooked midday meal, available every day at a very reasonable cost. As we were struggling financially, my mother was relieved to know I could have a very filling meal every day.

At home in our cramped apartment things were very difficult, and over the next couple of years, life became even worse. My father was killed in a car accident in Ireland. My sister, Irene, and her husband came to live with us, and shortly after they arrived, Irene developed severe and debilitating rheumatoid arthritis. My mother was also stricken with the same disease in the following year.

When I look back now, I cannot be certain of the exact timing of these catastrophic events. All I know is that by the time I was seventeen, my mother and sister were very ill. I watched with horror the extreme helplessness of my sister, and the onset of the severe physical crippling that was to progressively worsen over the years. I was terrified. It seemed as if we were all caught in some awful nightmare from which we could not awaken. My mother was very embittered and full of repressed rage, and she ruled the household with an iron will. We were not allowed to let down or collapse into emotions; feelings must be held in check at all costs. She was still angry with my father, of course, and when he died, she refused to go to his funeral. Nor did she allow any of the rest of us to do so—indeed, we were all forbidden to mourn him and his passing in any noticeable way.

When I was sixteen, I was withdrawn from school and had to begin to work to contribute to the family's financial well being. I also helped to care for my sister's two young children, who were born in quick succession and who also lived with us. Some two years after they were born, Irene's husband left her, and she struggled along with great courage, ill as she was, with help from all of us. My mother continued to go to church, where she lit candles and prayed for the strength to endure. Steeped in the dogma of the church, my mother was utterly persuaded by the model of the good, self-sacrificing female, the woman who asks for nothing for herself, and who endures all. She passed this unlivable doctrine on to my sister, who took its destructive message to heart. "Offer up your suffering to God, and know you will be rewarded in heaven"—that was the promise. A woman's task was to suffer in silence; it was a woman's lot to suffer. Did not God say to Eve, "I will intensify the pangs of your childbearing; in pain shall you bring forth children. Yet your urge shall be for your husband, and he shall be your master. For you are dust, and to dust you shall return." This vision of the fallen nature of female sexuality, and the torturous atonement one must make for a life so steeped in sin, twisted and distorted the lives of my mother and my sister, nor did I escape its corrosive influence.

As a young woman in such an environment, I was, of course, carefully watched and highly constrained both socially and sexually, a surveillance that merely deepened my feelings of loneliness and desperation. At last, however, I managed to find friends at work, and I joined a drama group that introduced me to improvisational movement, theatre, and music, including my first exposure to *The Planets*, by Holtz. This music with its glorious, moody, and dramatic tones matched my turbulent pent-up feelings. As a part of the drama group, I was able to act out various of my conflicting emotions. This was very cathartic and I loved every minute in the dramatic space, for it appealed to and allowed me to make something of my passionate nature. I was encouraged to let things out, not to hold them in. In the few years before my twentieth birthday, I managed to travel to Europe, Austria, Germany and France. I met and made friends with foreign exchange students, and began to dream of a world that was beyond the painful confines of our narrow home.

When I think of these years of my adolescence and emerging adulthood, and all of the trauma that was happening around me, I am tempted to refer to them as the years B.C., meaning Before Consciousness, particularly before feminist consciousness and before spiritual consciousness. The events all around me were so catastrophic, so shattering, that I was barely staying afloat.

I spent six years in Devon, during which time, as I've related, a number of challenging and major life-changing events occurred: there was my father's sudden death, my sister's marriage, the onset of her illness, the birth of her two children, the onset of my mother's illness, and all of this on top of the simple daily struggles of a marginalized immigrant family. I felt trapped and powerless before these events. They threatened to sweep me into a maelstrom of helplessness and despair and, buoyed by my brief escapes with friends, I decided I had to get out of the zone of my family's misfortune before I got caught in it for good. I agonized about how to break the news that I had decided to leave to my mother. I wanted to try to make a better life, to try things out on my own. My eldest sister, Lynn, was far away in Canada; I could go to her for a start. I felt an enormous sense of both guilt and relief when I finally told my mother that I was leaving. She did not protest, but I knew she felt very sad because I was her youngest child and a girl who could have helped her. Leaving her felt like a huge betrayal. All the same, I felt I had to go. My departure was as inevitable as the others' had been. Unknown to me, it was a very wounded self that I took with me to the new world.

I applied for and received landed immigrant status, and left England on April 20th 1967. I was twenty years old, and filled with hope and terror. Strong-willed and independent, I was determined to escape to a new life in Canada. I was unaware of the quantity of undeclared baggage I was carrying as I began this new stage in my life's journey. Intent upon the freedom and adventure of my new life, I did not realize that escape is not always accomplished once one walks away physically. Deep inside myself, I carried the terrible constraints, pains, repressions, and judgments of my old life; they were as sewn into me as my love of beauty, my passion, and curiosity. And *all* of these things would shape what I could do in my new home, how I would grow, who I would become.

The Land of The Free

I'm not sure if I thought that Canada would be the land of the free, but I am sure that I hoped it would be. Those who flee a difficult past to a new geography always hope their new country will bring freedom. And while the move to Canada was scary, and a part of me was fearful and full of self-doubt, another part of me was brave and fearless: my survivor self. I had nothing to lose, I thought; things couldn't have been much worse anywhere else. There was, so I heard, lots of work in Canada. And I could stay with my sister until I got established. What more did I need? This last plan, however, did not work out so well.

Lynn lived in a suburb of Montreal, Pointe-Claire, where houses and shops, all drawn from the same plan, and ringed about by square lawns and parking lots, crowded upon one another. I could not get used to this space that was neither urban nor rural. I got a job in a local shopping mall, but I hated its bland characterlessness. By June, I had escaped again; I moved downtown to a rooming house on Peel Street, just off Sherbrooke. I loved it! Montreal was a delightful, lively city; the French atmosphere reminded me of Europe and made me feel less lonely and more at home.

That first summer on my own was a wonderful adventure. I loved my room in that old house with its folding wooden shutters. Once I had arranged my few treasured possessions around me, I felt an intense sense of freedom, a huge feeling of relief. I had escaped a dire fate, I just knew it! I threw myself into experiencing the beauty of the city and making my way on my own. Of course, as a young woman who had left school early, I had no training or skills of any kind. Luckily for me, however, I eventually did find work at Expo 67, that huge international extravaganza which turned Montreal into an exciting city of fun and opportunity. My new residence and my work at Expo 67 also brought me into contact with the various lifestyles and experiences of other immigrants in Montreal in the sixties.

In the rooming house where I lived, there were two young men from Poland on my floor, and, in the basement, a young woman my age from England. We became fast friends. I remember the first time I met Pam, she was wearing a Marks and Spencer nylon housecoat, and she had giant rollers in her hair, of the sort that we used to straighten our hair in the sixties. She was from Liverpool, the home of the Beatles. She had lovely brown eyes, chestnut brown hair, and a soft, lilting voice. We hit it off instantly.

Interesting to me was the fact that Pam seemed to be angry a lot. She worked as a secretary, in those days when women secretaries were the housewives of offices. They bought and served the coffee; they were often expected to deal with the personal domestic requirements of the (naturally male) boss or supervisor. Blatant sexual harassment was common; if you wanted to keep your job, there was no recourse or space to protest. Pam often came home from work cursing and swearing under her breath; she would slam doors and kick garbage bins. Most of the time she was angry about work and angry with men. We had no social analysis in those days to help us sort out what was wrong, where and why. We simply realized it was unfair that women had so little overt political or social power and were so often so badly treated.

When Pam and I got down in the dumps and missed home, we would have a few drinks and listen to the latest music: Leonard Cohen, Bob Dylan, the Beatles, and Joan Baez. Folk music was what we liked best. Sometimes we got together with the Polish guys, who also felt marginalized as they searched for work and status in this new country. We had long and laboured conversations in broken English, interspersed with lots of laughter.

My first job, once I had my new place, was with a real estate company of dubious origin, which had set up an office in the Windsor Hotel by the train station. They offered free dinners to tourists who would listen to a presentation on land for sale in Florida. It was a great and familiar scam, which I naively aided and abetted. My job was to convince tourist couples to accept the dinner invitations I was handing out, and get them into the hotel. The salesman would do the rest of the talking and the pitch. Of course, as it turned out, the land for sale was the proverbial swampland in Florida, and so my job did not last long. Someone must have blown the whistle on the operation, because one morning when I walked into the office, everything and everyone had packed up and gone. In the end, this was a happy circumstance for me for it was time to move on to a better and more interesting job.

Expo 67 was in full swing, and I was dying to be involved. I met a girl who worked there who looked like a Viking princess. She had long, silver blond hair and pale creamy skin. She wore Indian clothing: long skirts and exotic jewelry. I remember that she had a wonderful cloak made out of Astrakhan fur. I was enchanted by everything about her. She introduced me to an Indian family who operated a boutique at Expo, and life suddenly got more interesting. I worked in the boutique and became close friends with the family. Fascinated by this exposure to yet another culture, I befriended the daughter, who was amazed at my freedom, as she was always under the watchful eye of her father and brothers. Under the influence of my new friends, I accumulated all sorts of Indian clothes and jewelry, and was suddenly, newly, excitingly fashionable. It seemed as if the whole world were opening up before me.

When Expo ended, all too soon, I had to get a steady job. It was a challenge to find something interesting, with so little formal training. Pam's experiences made me grateful that I lacked the office skills to make an effective secretary. No doubt I would have caused mayhem in any office where I worked had I been possessed of the requisite skills, for I had strong sense of justice and was enraged by and vocal about the subjugation of women. I looked in the *Montreal Star* and found an ad for a "child care worker" at an orphanage with training on the job. I went for an interview and discovered that the job was at a place that had formerly been an orphanage run by Catholic nuns. Under pressure of modernization from the government, new methods of psychiatric treatment were introduced, and the orphanage was in the process of being turned into a residential treatment center for children from broken homes. But the nuns were still doing the hiring. What an ironic twist of fate: there I was, not only back to the Catholic Church again, but more or less rescued by it. I was immediately given a job, for I was just the person to hire—a good Catholic Irish convent-educated girl. Indeed, irony aside, the job was good luck for me. The sisters were very kind and generous. They helped to train me, and looked after me in all sorts of important and tangible ways. They gave me furniture and bedding for my apartment, and nice old bookcases and chairs from the ancient Gothic building that they were vacating. They took me into the fold so to speak, and for the next three years, I embarked on an intense and life-changing work experience.

Again, at the treatment center, I worked with other immigrants like myself. The staff was mostly comprised of young draft dodgers from the States, but also included a young male social worker from England, a male social worker from New Delhi, and a young French woman from Montreal. When I look back now, I realize what an important step this new job was in my evolution. I was working with severely traumatized children who had suffered physical, sexual and emotional abuse. The work was exhausting on every level. The children, very angry and at the same time very sad, would often act out. In the old orphanage, this sort of acting out had been controlled by old-fashioned ways of behaviour modification: discipline, threat of privation and other punishments. Now, in the new treatment center, there was great focus on chemical intervention: the new psychiatric tool most often used to control the children's behaviour was Ritalin. In retrospect, it is hard to figure out which was the lesser of the two evils, old fashioned disciplinary tools, or new modes of psychiatric behaviour control.

Many of the children we saw were incest survivors, and enormously confused. And although I had had similar experiences, I was unable truly to relate to the upheavals and emotional trauma caused by sexual abuse in the children we saw. I could not face my own history then either. Luckily, I was not expected to analyze or treat the children in my charge. My job was to ensure the smooth running—if possible—of their daily lives, to make sure that they got up, got dressed, had their meals, got to school, did their chores, and kept their rooms in order with minimal fighting or harm to themselves and to others. This last task, of course, was the most difficult, because these children were angry and nobody wanted to enter into or to work with that anger. I also organized games and playtimes with the children.

First Awakening

I worked at the treatment center for three years, and then, having saved much of my earnings, I decided to make another big change. I left my job and moved out of the city onto a farm near Huntington, Quebec. I had always loved the country and preferred green spaces to the city. But, in making the move that I did, I also became a part of an idealistic movement of the early 1970s which involved the embrace of communal living, the glorification of nature, the search for alternate routes to meaningful living and well-being, and the revaluing of physical labour. In short, I became a part of the hippie movement "back to the land." I decided that I needed to make a change. I was very worn out from my work at the center, utterly burnt out. And I had become involved in a serious relationship with a man I had met. My instincts told me I needed to take time off, to think about our relationship, and make some decisions about my life. The promised peace and quiet of country life seemed to be the perfect antidote.

But things did not quite work out that way. My expectations were that I would live in quiet serenity, maybe gardening, certainly walking and horseback riding, as in the summer the farm was a riding camp. But right from the start, life on the farm was not what I expected. The owner of the place was a wild, macho Hungarian, with a definite predilection for seducing every young woman with whom he came into contact. His wife too sought out other company, if of a spiritual nature, and the farm soon became the haven for an avant-garde of artists, political activists, hippies, filmmakers and writers. Alternately engaged and bemused by the events all around me, I was blown away by the varieties and quantities of drugs that seemed to be floating around in our country paradise; these included some wonderful mescaline, which became my drug of choice, and great windowpane acid. Suddenly, I was not simply introduced to the drug culture of the psychedelic era, but utterly surrounded by it.

Despite my surroundings, however, I remained quite cautious about when and with whom I took drugs. My childhood had taught me that I must protect myself, that I must not leave myself vulnerable in social situations. Above all, I was quite wary of making myself too vulnerable with men who I did not know well. It was the period in which the so-called "sexual revolution" was in full swing; women were expected to "put out" without any hassles and everything that happened was cool and groovy. But, perhaps because I had been so sexually traumatized as a child, and because I was wary, perhaps also because I was very proud and insisted on having a large zone of respect around myself, I did not find it cool and groovy to sleep around—I was definitely more selective. By then, too, I was beginning to get in touch with a part of myself which surfaced in intimate relationships, and which I found very disquieting. As soon as I got involved with someone, I seemed to turn into a clingy, dependent person, which I hated. No doubt this was aided by the fact that I always fell for men who were not emotionally available. Men who thought I was great and fell in love with me and were emotionally present to me, bored me; I quickly found fault in anyone interested in truly making a relationship with me. Indeed, I eagerly pursued, and then married, a man who was for the most part aloof and emotionally unreachable.

Later, of course, through the years of my counselor-training and my extensive reading, I came to see very clearly how such a pattern plays out. If we have been abandoned, and that is our most profound and forceful experience, then we seek out and choose those who will abandon us. We are compelled to repeat the pattern of our pain in an unconscious effort to heal the original injury: "If only I can make him love me, then I can become whole; the wound of my abandonment will be healed."

In my case, as I repeated the pattern of reaching for someone emotionally unreachable, my sense of abandonment or my fear of it did not leave me, and I felt myself falling into a very dependent and insecure state. In this state, I went through agonies of feeling rejected, unloved, powerless, and I was quite at a loss to know from which part of me such emotions emerged. When I was footloose and on my own, I felt strong, fearless, and full of adventure. Then to my horror, in a relationship, I turned into a clinging helpless victim.

I went to the farm to try to heal myself of this puzzling and distressing love-cycle. That did not happen, but I was exposed to the drug scene, as well as a number of new ideas and thoughts about how to live. Now I realize that these experiences were like seeds, which, long dormant, suddenly flower in unexpected and utterly unrelated ways many years later.

Up to that point, I had done very little reading on altered states of consciousness, save for Aldous Huxley's *The Doors of Perception*. And when I arrived at the farm, as a woman who was initially quite cautious about drugs, I found myself often on the sidelines as a caretaker when people dropped acid; I looked out for those who had bad trips, cooked, and tried to help others patch up relationships. But eventually I did my own experimenting with altered states, and I discovered that of all of the hallucinogens on offer at the farm, mescaline was my favorite. It was smooth, came on easy— mostly high and light; it definitely shifted one into alternate zones. On mescaline, I experienced a blissful awareness of being "part of it all." Such states were not always easy: heightened awareness could also be terrifying, as unexpectedly memories and events from the past or the present loomed up before you in emotional technicolour. However joyous, frightening, or moving, I often found these experiences of altered states also deeply religious—in the sense of knowing that one was part of a larger cosmic plan, a supreme intelligence or order. Such feelings were awesome and numinous. This sense of being in the presence of something holy particularly pertained to my experiences of the world of nature when I was high. Very often, in such a state, I would wander in the fields, laying myself down in the river, and letting the stream of water wash over me; I would look at the rocks breathing and the trees dancing. I remember one time, on acid, seeing streams of energy radiating from everything, I murmured to myself, 'everything is energy, everything is light.'

While positive reflections on the meaningful quality of hallucinogenic insights are no longer popular in this, our contemporary anti-drug, era, I believe that my experience on hallucinogens opened some important doors to my own self- and other-understanding, consciousness, and spiritual growth. In those days, in the early seventies, as I soon discovered when I began to seek more information on the experiences I was having, a number of scientists, thinkers, and psychologists were doing research on altered states of consciousness and writing about it. They included Richard Alpert (Ram Dass), Timothy Leary, Alan Watts and Stan Grof. Indeed, Grof's research, which he wrote about in *Realms of the Human Unconscious*, argued that the bad trips that so many of us sometimes experienced on these mind-altering drugs were a consequence of the fact that, under the influence of the drugs, we often re-experienced repressed traumatic material which we had split off from. Bringing such unresolved experiences into consciousness again is always terrifying and risky, but it is also sometimes, in a therapeutic setting, the first step towards healing. Of course we, in our recreational use of hallucinogens, did not have the understanding or skills to deal productively and progressively with such fragile states. We could simply try not to abandon one another as, alone, sometimes we dropped into the abysses of psychotic or near-psychotic conditions. Still, high as the price sometimes was, most of us were prepared to risk the dangers of the drugs that we took in order also to experience their glories, those transcendental, deeply mystical, transpersonal states that Grof also wrote about, in which, suddenly, you caught a glimpse of the divine, and were caught up in its embrace.

My experiences on the farm opened up and changed my life in some quite startling ways. That period was quite a turbulent, exciting time and now when I think back on it, I realize that my experiences there prompted an enormous shift in my consciousness. Ultimately, I could say, they helped me to bring into focus what would become, as the years went on, an increasingly important spiritual focus. But first, before I began again to pursue this transformative spiritual dimension, came my years of social activism in the woman's movement. I did, as I've mentioned, marry. We had a child, left the farm, and moved to rural Nova Scotia to try to buy land. We had heard, through friends, that farmland was affordable in Nova Scotia, and I was interested in finding a quiet country environment where we could raise our child. Although the marriage did not last this new experiment, I loved Nova Scotia, and put down roots there. Once more I was by the ocean, surrounded by breathtaking scenery, not far from Antigonish, a university town. It was an idyllic setting, peaceful and stimulating. Many things were possible. I made new friends, built strong community ties, and, after the break-up of my marriage, made a lasting and sustaining, healthy relationship with a man, who helped me to raise my eldest son, and with whom I had two further marvelous children, a son and a daughter.

Consciousness-Raising

My interests and activities, in the next twenty years after I moved to Nova Scotia, were fueled by a quest for justice, particularly in the area of feminism and women's rights. No doubt, in my initial openness to and interest in women's rights, I was inspired by my childhood experience of the deep shame and powerlessness of the women around me. Happily for me, I had gotten the message early on that women were my allies, that we might build trust with each other instead of competing for men, that we were intelligent, strong, fierce, caring, creative and far more resourceful than any of the images of us everywhere presented in our culture.

Over those years, and particularly after the end of my marriage, I embarked on a journey to restore myself to myself as a strong and powerful loving woman. The key thread in this restoration of body and spirit was my link with other women, particularly our activism and our reclamation of the divine. Over the course of ten years, from the mid- seventies to the mid-eighties, I read through the extensive new research on early Goddess religions, and another piece fell into place for me. Finding the Goddess helped me to heal from the shame and bodily self-hatred that I had carried with me since my childhood. Over the same period of time, I had the unique experience of gathering regularly with a small group of women, and using ritual to celebrate our sacredness and the sacredness of the earth. During these years, I worked in the peace movement and helped to support the opening of a battered women's shelter in the community. Indeed, I worked as a crisis counselor in the shelter for several years and I was also involved in the opening of a women's resource center. All these were radical acts in a socially conservative Roman Catholic community.

It was not easy to be working on such politically charged issues in a community that maintained a great deal of denial around sexuality and women's issues. I had gotten used to controversy and was not unused to challenging old assumptions and outdated stereotypes, but still, I faced my own challenges in dealing with these questions as well. Was I a bad person if I acted from my own concerns and feelings, rather than forever submerging myself in other's needs and concerns? Was it wrong and selfish to want to develop that part of me that I could call my *self* in the first place? Why couldn't I just be happy being a mother and get on with my life, rather than balking and protesting at every sign of the diminishment of women, on every level and in every arena, political, economic, personal and spiritual? There must be something more to my life than simply getting on, a purpose, a higher calling. In time this questioning translated into a spiritual hunger, and not simply a hunger for social justice.

With each step, each struggle, my understanding grew, and I began to have a sense of my calling, of the meaningful work that I could do, with and for myself, and others. In 1986, I returned to school, to St. Francis Xavier University, where I took a diploma program in adult education. Choosing to do my field project on "Women and Self-Esteem," I developed a series of workshops on women's self-esteem. In the following years, repeatedly conducting these workshop sessions with numerous different groups provided me with significant evidence of the enormous conflict many women feel when they try to develop a "self." Again and again I witnessed the split, the guilty war, the impossible resolution between selfhood and sacrifice in many women's lives. The stories I heard in my workshops, the situations I saw in the battered women's shelter and in the women's center reconfirmed the centrality of this question of sacrifice to women's struggles for self-determination and self-esteem. We were not as far from the days of my Irish Catholic childhood as perhaps many of us thought.

CHAPTER II

A Call to Change

Having gotten this far, now in my early forties, a drama was about to unfold which would throw me into a new phase of change and self-growth. How many times in life must we heed a call to change, or recognize an opportunity that requires us to embark on an adventure that leads toward the unknown? What conditions are required to set the stage that will enable us to start on such a journey, that will allow us to be open and receptive to the powers of change and the influence of guidance in our lives? Such calls to change are difficult to answer, above all when they look as if they will cause major upheaval, force us to re-evaluate how we view the world, even reality itself, or push us to expand our boundaries and review our most cherished self-imposed limitations.

Such a call to change happened to me in 1990. It was not the first time I had embarked on a journey into the unknown; after all, I had gone from England to Canada, and, even earlier, at fourteen, left my childhood home in Ireland to move to England. The former was self-chosen, of course, the latter a situation of parental decision.

The decision to "change" in 1990, however, to answer the call to embark on a new path of self-discovery, happened at a time of great personal crisis. The events that occurred—which I will describe in some detail in this chapter—precipitated a spiritual awakening, an opening to a different reality or state of consciousness. Roberto Assagioli, an Italian psychoanalyst and psychiatrist, a younger contemporary of Freud and Jung, described these states or experiences of spiritual consciousness as the "true source or essence of being" or "life in greater abundance." Arguing that psychiatry and psychoanalysis in their normative practice ignored the importance of the spiritual dimension, Assagioli began to publish papers on the principles and theories of a transpersonal or spiritually attuned psychology in the first two decades of the twentieth century. In 1926, he opened his first therapeutic treatment center and training program in Rome, the Instituto di Cultura e Terapia Psichica: the Institute of Psychic Culture and Therapy. Psychosynthesis, as his approach was called in English, was born.

In the course of a spiritual awakening, according to Assagioli,

> *very often there is a sense of enlightenment, a new unearthly light which transfigures the external world and a light which reveals a new beauty. It illuminates the inner world, throws light on problems and doubts and dispels them. It is the intuitive light of a higher consciousness.*

Such a sense of spiritual awakening can be seen as the birth of new being within us; often it is accompanied by a sense of renewal and regeneration. Of course this new being within us has always been there, but it seems as if we have to be born to it anew— this notion of rebirth is often referred to in the New Testament. We are being reborn to a part of us that is already within us: "Behold, the Kingdom of heaven is within you. So we awaken to our divine nature, to god/ess within us."

A NEW BEING, BORN WITHIN US!

Exciting news, but at the time that it began to occur, I had no idea that this new being was being born within me. Indeed, it seemed then as if my world were falling apart. It felt as if I were, quite literally, stopped in my tracks; my forward momentum slowed; physically and psychically, the way that I had been was grinding to a halt. I remember clearly the sense of speed and agitation that ruled my life before the onset of my illness. I was forty-three years old, in abundant physical health, and in many respects, quite unaware of the speediness of my inner and outer worlds. After nearly two decades of feminist and social activist work, I suddenly lost my forward-looking energy and fell into a state of burn-out and disillusionment. For years I had struggled against the powers that be, against institutions and ideologies that valued and privileged men's lives over women's, male development and freedom over female development and freedom. For years I had walked, talked, breathed, eaten, and lived the effort to critique and dismantle the thrall of old patriarchal attitudes in our lives, and then, at my work in the Battered Women's Shelter, a personal battle with a co-worker made me feel as if everything was lost. I felt that I had been deceived and betrayed. How could this have happened there, in that safe space? The forces that we were fighting were supposed to be outside, out there in the faulty world as men ran it, not in each other, or so I thought. Now of course I understand that the sense of betrayal and deception that I had was intimately bound up with my own deep need to be in control of my way of seeing and experiencing the world, the right way, of course! All of my judgements fell from the vantage point of this very controlled vision I had of how the world should be; I was righteousness and looked in judgement on others who were less right than I. The urgency to change the world justified my refusal to look inward; it justified my speediness, even the speed and harshness of my judgements. But in the course of this battle with my co-worker, my views were called into question, and not simply by others, but, suddenly, crucially, by me, myself. After the awful fallout, I scraped myself together a bit, and realized that it was time for a change. I decided to take a year off to enrol in Stillpoint, a New Age Massage school in Massachusetts where there was a strong focus on spiritual and personal growth.

And so, in the summer of 1989, I prepared to leave my family and friends in Nova Scotia, the community where I had lived for 15 years, and move to Massachusetts. I remember having a conversation with a woman friend that summer, also a feminist activist, about the direction my life was taking. "In the final analysis I don't think we have control of what happens in our lives," I said as I went on to explain how I had planned for a year to be able to go to this school. How I had saved enough money to pay for tuition, and tried to prepare my three children for the changes and adjustments of a year away from me in which they would have to rely on their father for most of their care-taking. My friend, surprised and indignant, replied, "What do you mean you don't have control? If you believe that then how can you believe in social change? Why bother doing all this work?!"

I responded, "I have prepared in every way possible to spend this year in massage school but anything could happen. My partner could have an accident, my son could fall out of a tree; anything could happen that would in an instant collapse all my well laid plans." We argued this point for a while in good humour, neither of us convincing the other. As the time of my departure grew closer, I often found myself thinking, "This experience will change me and change my life." I had no idea how much it would, nor how profoundly that change would differ from my expectations.

I had decided, following that disastrous episode at work, that I would set myself the goal of letting go of control in my life. What exactly did that mean? I don't think that I knew much then about what such a goal would mean, but I had begun to perceive how controlling I was in my daily life with my partner and our children—even the physical space around me had to be the way I dictated it should. I hated change: I would not allow my partner to alter anything about the house, and I remember musing to myself as I looked around before I left, "I really have no control now over what he or the children do or change in this house or in their routines." Now of course I see how utterly unaware I was of the profound changes about to take place, and the truth in my insistence that in the final analysis we don't have total control seems uncanny.

I said goodbye to my partner and my three children, knowing that my heart was very protected; I did not allow myself to feel the pain or loss of leaving them, of missing them. A familiar response for me when separated from loved ones had been to deny my feelings and forge ahead, forcing myself through sheer power of will to get through whatever was before me. I moved into a house in Northampton, Massachusetts, where the owners were quiet and quite laidback. Everything there, from my view, was slowed down. I proceeded, in my indomitable fashion, to try to speed things up; I was a whirlwind of cleaning, straightening, hauling, lawn-mowing, care-taking activity. In this household were a small baby girl and an eleven-year-old boy. I rented a room on the first floor of the house, which was to be my haven throughout the course of the coming events, events that halted the flow of my life and shook the foundations of my faith in life, in God and in justice.

Shortly after I arrived, I had written in my journal:

September 2, 1989
Saturday, Northampton, Massachusetts
Here for four days, happily settled in this pretty room with my lovely Mexican blanket on the bed, my goddess picture on the wall, all my little things around me. Sage through the room today —to clear out the energies and purify the space. I can't believe I am here and miles away from all my family. Saying goodbye was hard.
It was the first day of my period and I wanted to sit down and cry my eyes out. I did for a few minutes but I am here—alive, healthy, eating very well. Dying to start school and get into it — 40 students this year!

In another diary, my "Red Book," a notebook which travelled with me to school everyday, I wrote:

Stillpoint is an amazing place. It seems that it is a place where all the spiritual and healing things I have thought about can be used, talked about, and lived, with complete acceptance and validity.

I had a deep longing to learn about healing, to learn how healing takes place, and to better understand the connections between body, mind, spirit and emotions. Watching the tragedy of my sister and my mother falling ill, caught in the grip of the crippling disease—arthritis —which destroyed their lives, informed my longing very profoundly. Having fled England and established my own life in Canada, far away from their misery, nevertheless, I was compelled to return to the deep questions, which I had guiltily fled, provoked by their illnesses. Now in my forties, I suddenly wanted desperately to understand how and why these things happened. What was the meaning of illness? What could we learn from these experiences of breakdown? Most of all how could one learn to get better, by which, of course, I meant, return to health and wholeness. My view of health then was embodied by the person I was at the beginning of that school year: active, energetic, ready to meet any challenge with the knowledge of my sound good health and robust nature. But what I hadn't considered in that picture, although I sometimes felt its loss, was the role that a spiritual life might play in health and in healing. Health could not be a matter of one's physical fitness alone.

On November 22, 1989, I was called home to England. I was sitting down to write an anatomy exam when my eldest son, Jesse, called Stillpoint and asked me to phone my nephew in England. My heart stopped and I could feel my stomach tighten into a knot. I went to the office and put a call through to England. The news was not good. My older sister Irene was in the hospital, very weak and close to death, and I should come back as quickly as possible if I wanted to see her. In a moment, everything became confused and unreal. Somehow I booked a flight for the next day. I purchased an open ticket, which allowed me to travel on my return whenever I wished. The school was very supportive, telling me I could sit again for my exams when I returned.

No accident perhaps but it was around this time that I began to experience severe pain in my shoulder. The day I booked my flight, I was in a great deal of pain so I quickly made an appointment with a chiropractor recommended by the school. When I walked into his office, I burst into tears. I was in so much physical pain, and I was so upset and depressed about my sister's illness, that I collapsed on the chiropractor's table and poured out my anguish and pain. Underlying all of my more obvious worries were fear and guilt about the costs of going to England—I worried about running out of money. I was on a very strict budget at school, a budget that I tried to supplement by working to clean the office space there. A thousand dollars for an open ticket to England would make a huge hole in the money I had saved for school. Things were going down hill fast. The chiropractor did some very delicate cranial sacral work, and generously deferred payment till I returned from England.

What I did not realize at the time, and what none of the many practitioners who worked with me over the next months were aware of, was the fact that I too had begun to develop rheumatoid arthritis—that dreaded family disease that had so crippled my sister. As a new mother, at the age of 23, she had been diagnosed. Then, when her second child was born not long afterward, she could barely lift him out of his crib. I was in my mid-teens then, and watched the devastation wrought by this disease with horror. My sister was put on a strong dose of steroids, Prednisone, a drug which she remained on for more than 20 years. The side affects of this drug included the disintegration of bone tissue. Her spine eventually became like a honeycomb or sponge, the veins, and thus circulation, broke down in her legs, causing gangrene to set in. Both legs had to be amputated. Over the years, she had had both hips replaced, knees, hands and wrists: many major operations, all the while trying to raise her two children on her own. Her husband left her; he could neither bear nor handle her illness.

At around the same time, my mother developed both rheumatoid and osteo-arthritis in her early fifties: the tragedy was thus twofold. Both women were caught in the grip of this vicious illness, while as a teenager, I stood by feeling terror and powerlessness. I just wanted to get away from it all, away from the pain and guilt and apparent helplessness of our household. Having fled an abusive husband with her two youngest children, my mother felt that her illness was a curse on her for her sinfulness, her disobedience, her daring to break out of the mould of the good Catholic woman, to leave marriage and find a life for herself. Her terrible guilt was exacerbated by the fact that my father had been killed two years after her departure in an awful car accident. My mother would not return to Ireland for the funeral, nor were we permitted to talk about it or him or to mourn any loss we might have felt. My sister, who deeply cared for my father, was thus denied her grief, and she carried the guilt of knowing that she had denied his request to see her just weeks before he died. Three months after his death, pains started in her back during her first pregnancy, and in a matter of months, her world fell apart.

It was my sister who took the phone call informing the family that my father had been killed. Within weeks her illness started; my mother's illness started soon after. Both women suffered from profound emotional pain and guilt, which no doubt affected them on every level of their being. I began to wonder, was the extent of this emotional pain and shock so far reaching as to make manifest illness and pain on a physical level—or at least, to contribute to that physical illness? What was the connection between emotional and physical pain for these two women? What was the connection between emotional and physical pain in the circumstances of the onset of my illness? What part did this thread of abandonment and guilt play in all our lives? Did I, like my mother, feel I was being punished by daring to have a life of my own, by placing my needs above others? Surely, taking a year such as I had decided I would at Stillpoint was a *selfish* thing for a woman to do.

I had chosen to live in the country, to raise my children with healthy food and in a clean environment. So far I had been rewarded with abundant health, a close loving mutual relationship with the man I loved, the father of my children. Our three children were healthy and happy. We were indeed very blessed, and I was very aware that we lived a privileged life. Every day we celebrated life on our piece of land in beautiful Nova Scotia; I was acutely conscious of how fortunate I was. Yet like many others, I took my health for granted and I believed in the goodness and healthfulness of my lifestyle, which was, in large part, why I never suspected that when the pains in my shoulder started, I had arthritis. Indeed, it never entered my mind. No, it seemed like I had got away with it, with something that my mother and sister had not. I had made my great escape to Canada, and along with it, a fine new life. I had taken *control* of my life, fled sentiments and sensations of terror and powerlessness, of a woman's helplessness and servitude to patriarchal church morality.

Now twenty years later, I was boarding a plane to fly to England to be at my sister's deathbed. But she did not die then. Once again, she proved her indomitable spirit and survived; she continued to live at home with round-the-clock health care. Over the years, I had watched my sister struggle with this relentless disease, and it was a great source of fear and sadness to me. I always felt so powerless when I was with her— and so relieved to come back to Canada to the safety of my healthy lifestyle!

Soon after I returned from England, I realized that my sister had survived once again because she was not ready to die. When I had first arrived and walked into the hospital with her daughter, we quickly realized that her total despondency was in a large part due to her fear and hatred of hospitals. I stayed with my sister long enough to help her daughter have her transferred back home and settled with the nursing care she needed. I returned to Canada for Christmas with bad shoulder pain. I was concerned but felt my pain would easily get sorted out when I got back to my chiropractor in Massachusetts.

I returned to school in January, and remained in close touch with my sister, who was still struggling to stay alive. My heart was very heavy. I had written in my diary on January 28, 1990:

> *I am feeling despondent tonight in my little room, feeling the weight of the world on my shoulders— the money I owe for Stillpoint, the money I spent in England. My shoulder is still bad. I can't do my work. What is it? Is it my denial of the guilt I feel over using some of the family money to be here? I just had a letter from the Canadian Women's Foundation—no luck there for money. I want so desperately to get better. What do*

I need to do to take this weight off my shoulders, to get the guilt off my back? No it won't work that way; I have to let it go. I wish I could shake off this depression.

When I read this entry now, I recall the depth of my misery and depression, my fear, I did not know what was going on. Everything seemed so unfair! So unjust! I certainly did not deserve this so why was it happening to me? All I had wanted to do was help others. I felt a deep sense of failure, a sense that would become familiar to me as time went on.

Meanwhile, back in Nova Scotia, my partner and children were very worried about me. I tried to make light of what was happening and insisted that the chiropractic work was helping me. By now, however, I had tried several chiropractors and was also working with an acupuncturist. My diet was extremely healthy—yet I was progressively getting worse. Four things haunted me: guilt about money (this was, for me, as it is for so many, an old pattern developed when I was a child), a sense of failure or of being thwarted in my efforts, a deep fear of the unknown, and last but far from least, my old bugaboo, the terror of being out of control.

February 19, 1990
After days of intense pain, depression, anger, and frustration, I reached rock bottom and broke down in class. Janice worked on me, then I went to my chiropractor appointment. But I did not get my usual chiropractor. This new guy was so rough and invasive: after the session I freaked out and continued crying and let out the grief like unblocking a dam. I went home. Bev came in at 11pm and realized that if I did not get painkillers I would not sleep. She went to buy some. At midnight, I swallowed 2 and was out. The whole process was such a relief: to let down and let go; to realize that I don't have to hold it all in.

The goal I set for myself—to let go of control in my life—had manifested with more force and impact than I had anticipated. Several things happened at once: there were my sister's struggles to survive and my involvement in that process; there was my own physical crisis, not to mention my sense of loss in the long separation from my family; too, there was my persistent sense of failure and depression, and my inability to ask for help. As things got worse—and they did—I felt that every event was conspiring to disrupt my life and to block me from achieving my goals.

At school I could not do the required clinical massage work. In mid-February, my health deteriorated even further. The pains were now in my knees, ankles, and elbows; indeed, it felt as if they were moving around in my body. I could barely walk, and getting around at school was proving to be more and more difficult. On February 10, I noted in my diary what I had learned thus far from the crisis in my life and health:

A) I do not allow others to help me.
B) I feel more in control if I am the one helping.
C) I pride myself on being healthy and fit all of the time.
D) I block my feelings and my life energy.
E) I hold back the tension, fears, and anger that I feel.

Today was such a day of release. I stayed here in my room. I ate rice and vegetable broth, and continued to drink lots of water. I read and meditated, did yoga and affirmations. Tonight, I went and cleaned at the school offices.

During these early weeks in the progression of my illness, I tried various cleansing diets and juice fasts in an effort to detoxify my body. I meditated daily, and sometimes twice daily, working through important affirmations, trying desperately to turn my decline and pain around. I read several books on diets, fasting, and cleansing. I lost some weight and cleaned up my eating habits—no sugar, no caffeine!—but the pain and symptoms continued. I was beginning to learn a lot more than I had ever wanted to know about fear and vulnerability, and worse still, I was becoming very familiar with pain. I would not use any form of pain relief. But then the crisis suddenly became much worse.

Saturday, February 17, 1990

A dark day for me. I went to clean Steve Miller's office. I had awakened with a sore hand, all of the veins in the back of my hand hurt badly when I flexed my wrist. HORRORS, I thought, what's happening now— carpal tunnel syndrome? I looked it up in the Merck manual, but there was no way of knowing if that's what it was. Went to Holly's: she did some wonderful Feldenkreis work on my shoulders and arms, then I came home and noticed terrible pain in my left hip socket. I could barely walk and had to lift my foot to get into bed. Intense pain all night: I felt the crushing intensity of such bodily pain, and lay awake facing down all of my fears of disability. I can't walk, can't use my hands; my feet are swollen. What is this? Psychic and physical cleansing? Preparing me, challenging me, putting me through the fires. Can I trust, do I trust the universe and my body—the healing process where I am being challenged? In my weakness and lack of faith?

Sunday, February 18, 1990

All of my symptoms have subsided to varying degrees—my hand is better. My hip is 80% better. I am out of continual pain; I feel a lot better. I meditated, cleaned the house. Raised the massage table and called Maria to come for a massage; I pray and meditate, trust in god/ess.

Monday, February 19, 1990

Left hip locked. I spent all day in pain. I went to Dr. Boyden at 5:30. It will be my last visit to the chiropractors office as I am broke, flat out of money. He did another sacral iliac adjustment. I went home, but could not sleep. Chris called; he and the children are coming to visit on March 12th. We had a good chat; I went back to bed, but did not sleep all night.

I had an excellent chiropractor who was very puzzled by what was going on with me and no doubt wondered why he was not able to help me. When my partner Chris called, I could not tell him what was really going on, nor could I say how badly I was feeling.

March 4, 1990

I feel better, more myself tonight. I am

determined to be in good shape when Chris and the children arrive on Saturday. I hope they drive carefully. I feel better—HURRAH. I've got to start doing lots of massages soon.

March 17, 1990
Chris and the children left at six o'clock this morning. We had such a wonderful week. It was sunny and hot!! 70 degrees. I wanted so much to be better—and of course I had a flare-up in my left wrist and hand; it was <u>extremely</u> painful. I think it freaked Chris and Jesse out. The little ones did not notice it as much.

I still had not gotten the message and thought that the pain was caused by a hurt tendon—but what I was experiencing was an inflammatory response in my joints and tissues, no doubt about it.

It is raining tonight: a delightful sound. I am so glad to be on my own again to work on the many levels of my self-healing. I really believe most illness and disease stems from the spirit. I have to participate in raising my spiritual levels, to make a change in my life and my heart, soul and mind. I feel as if I am being tested as a potential healer. I am going through the fires. I am praying for guidance and seeking to restore harmony in whatever way I can. I am trying acupuncture; I am re-activating my crystal. I am working with diet, with vitamins; I am also working on releasing grief and looking at my sadness about my sister Irene. The healing waters, blue, light, cooling, and healing —drawn from the planetary life force—come to me again and teach me to listen, to be still and open.

When I look back at what I have written, I feel a great compassion for who I was then and how I struggled. There I was, steeped in New Age readings, books on healing, arguments that all illness stems from one's spiritual state. Of course, there is some truth to such arguments, but it was also true that I was genetically pre-disposed to get arthritis, and no amount of "purifying" my spirit could save me from the accidents of my genetic make-up. Unaware of the limits of my body, I read dozens of books on healing, books that argued that *you can heal your life if you try*. I read about how healers were often tested with illness to prove their readiness to do their work. Certainly, there is a measure of truth to such claims, but at the time, I felt that I had to heal myself of the entirety of my physical disease—or else I was a failure, which I suppose I was, according to the exacting, unwisdom of certain New Age standards. Now, too, when I read over the things that I wrote in March of 1990, I see evidence of a good deal of *magical thinking*—familiar enough to me during my childhood, but obviously I had kept it with me: If only I do all the right things—*if I am good enough,* this ailment, these bad things, will get better or go away. *I am praying for guidance and seeking to restore harmony*—how my heart goes out now to that person that I was! I was trying so hard to be a better person, to ward off all of the bad things that were happening to me. *If only I were good enough, I would cure myself!* I thought.

In the meantime, I tried every possible alternative healing method, anything but conventional medical treatment. The pain was awful; I do not know how I withstood it. Today, I imagine that my sedimentation rate, a measure deriving from a standard blood test, used to estimate the degree of arthritic inflammation and consequent joint damage, must have been close to a hundred. Of course, I still had no idea that what I was suffering from was arthritis. No doubt, even if I had known, that knowledge would not have made any difference, for I suspect I would have remained quite biased against using conventional medical drugs. I was very clear then: I would not have anything to do with conventional medicine; I had seen my sister suffer such catastrophic side-effects, that I was convinced that conventional approaches would not do me any good.

> *March 18, 1990*
>   *My feet have been very sore and swollen today, and my right thumb is extremely painful, hence this awful handwriting. I am ready for the end of these symptoms, I want to yell, scream Aaaah! Tomorrow, acupuncture at 8:30am. Chris called tonight; he sounded down in the dumps ; he really is fed up with*

being on his own. I must have faith —and hurry up my
healing.
'I believe in the sun even when it does not shine
I believe in love even when it is not shown.
I believe in God even when he does not speak.'
This message was scratched into a basement wall in
Germany during the time of the Holocaust!!! I must
have faith in healing, belief in God, in divine life force,
hope ever present.

I remember reading the passage about belief that I cited in *Love, Medicine and Miracles* by Bernie Siegel. Over and over again the same theme repeated itself in my thoughts and my writings: *if I believe enough—I will be healed.* What I did not realize then was that I might indeed be healed, but being healed might not include being cured of arthritis. Something was happening to me, in me, but it was perhaps not exactly what I thought would or should happen. As a part of my self-healing practice, I collected inspirational thoughts and statements about belief, statements like: *"He who believes in me shall be saved, and have ever-lasting life,"* that was the promise of Jesus Christ. If not exactly a call to the Christ of my childhood Catholicism, I did begin to hear the promise of everlasting life as a call to the recognition of the importance of a spiritual life, a life which transcends the illusion of this daily earthly life, which, of course, some consider to be all that there is.

There was so much pain in my life—physical pain, emotional pain, the pain of feeling abandoned, the pain of feeling as if I were a failure. These were all feelings that deepened when Chris called me in the middle of March from Nova Scotia, where I knew that it was still cold, still winter; it was the hardest season there, alone with the kids, out in the country, with no respite soon in sight. I felt that I had to hurry up my healing so that I could help him and everyone else out. Help everyone else? Wasn't that the image of the good selfless woman I imagined that I should be? As my mother had also believed about herself, secretly, I imagined that my illness was a punishment from God for my wrongdoing. If I had been a good self-sacrificing woman, if I had occupied the place that I was supposed to, then these bad things, this horrible pain, would not happen to me. I had not simply inherited a tendency to arthritis from my mother, but I had also inherited a host of damaging attitudes and beliefs. You became ill because of your *selfishness* and wrongdoing, or you became ill or met with misfortune because that was simply your cross to bear. For in bearing such a cross, we suffer in this life and are rewarded in heaven in the next. Thus I am sure that my mother believed that her own illness was a punishment for her selfishness, her wilfulness in leaving my father, and a cross she had to bear.

When I left my family then, my partner and children, and went to North Hampton—making the choice to support myself and my own personal growth over their wish to keep me near—I must have felt, somehow, despite the differences in the circumstances surrounding our actions, that I was repeating the pattern of my mother's life. My story shared certain features with hers—I was abandoning my family to search for my life. Certainly, I felt keenly the loss of a period of everyday life with my family, but I closed down those emotions as soon as I got started at Stillpoint. In the end, I see that I did exactly as I had been taught to do by my mother. I shut down my feelings of pain, and got on with the job once again, but in a new register, abandoning my self, turning my attention away from what was really going on, what was most important to me.

Life is suffering, said the Buddha. But, unlike in the Christian story that scripted my mother's despair, the suffering referred to by Buddhism is not imposed by a wrathful God. Rather, Buddhism suggests that what suffering we experience, we have created for ourselves in our profound resistance to change. Suffering is an experience common to us all on this earth, and nothing safeguards us from suffering of one kind or another: no belief system, no diet, no quantity of exercise or "correct" bodywork. The words I had taken from my reading of Bernie Siegel, the words scratched on the basement wall in Germany, echoed my sense of struggle, pain, hopelessness, despair, and abandonment. I wanted to cry out, to rant and rave and scream at the unfairness of everything that happened to me—yet I wanted to believe in God, even in my abandonment.

The next entry in my journal is not dated, but it repeats the themes I had been working over. The separation that I wanted to maintain between happiness, trust, faith and love, and pain is painfully clear.

> *If only I am good enough I will get better, bad things will not happen. I did a massage today with Mary; she talked about polarity and how wonderful it felt. She said how she trusted me and what marvellous hands I had. I am so happy - trust - faith - love. <u>And there is pain, of course.</u>*

I had done some energy work called polarity in the session that I wrote about—given the physical shape I was in, it was the only kind of massage work I could do then. When I had started massage school, I had very strong hands. I was used to doing enormous amounts of manual, outdoor work: digging and planting large gardens, splitting and stacking wood, sewing thick pieces of leather together with cord, and so on. And then, all of my strength evaporated, or so it seemed. It flowed through my hands, from my hands, like water.

Although I was in acute pain, I persisted in cleaning the office in order to pay for my acupuncture treatments. The sessions were very helpful and seem to initiate a lot of emotional release: I know I talked about my sister Irene a lot, because I was thinking about her constantly. I knew that she was struggling with dying, that she was trying to sort out when she would be able to let go and how. I was filled up with grief, which I was able to release in some measure during the course of my acupuncture sessions. That emotional release deepened my relationship with Irene. I began a series of nightly prayers and meditations for her; I sent her healing energy and love. Every night I lit a candle and thought about her; I prayed for her release into the light if she was ready.

Over the course of my year at Stillpoint, Irene and I became much closer. I had not known her well when we were both children in Ireland. Some years older than me, she had left home to work in England and gotten married. By the time I moved there with my mother and my brother, she seemed settled, grown-up. Then, when she became ill, her husband left her and she moved in with us, I had struggled to get away; I was in the process of growing up into my own life. Still, over the years, before my illness, we wrote one another frequently, sharing our love of literature and learning, and as time went on and my interest grew in health, healing, growth, and wholeness, we discussed all these topics. We seemed even then to have a soul connection. Because of her illness her life and movement had been curtailed—as far as working in the world went. Perhaps because of this, she particularly strongly supported and encouraged my goals in learning and in finding the work that I wanted to do. Indeed, a couple of years after I left Stillpoint, she not only whole-heartedly supported my desire to pursue training to become a Psychosynthesis therapist, but she also offered to pay my tuition fees, an offer which made all the difference, and, as we shall see, my training and present life possible.

As my illness progressed, Irene and I became guides and teachers for each other in this life, learning from and supporting each other's struggles in pursuit of freedom. I do not know what I would have done without her.

Meanwhile, in Massachusetts, spring progressed. So did my illness, and my healing, although I did not perceive that at the time.

> *March 21, 1990*
> *Spring: returning life—hard work, pain, confronting my monsters, consciously going through the agonies and despair. Today my feet are almost back to normal, my hands are a lot better, and also my knees, thank the goddess. I went to the nursing home in Leeds to do my field placement work; I sat with two old women and massaged their hands and feet and spent a humbling time sharing connection and loving energy with them. I was so grateful to be there and be of service in any small way. I will continue to pray, to be grateful for health, to seek inside myself for inner knowledge and strength, and to flush the*

*poisons of fear and self-despair out of my
psyche and all levels of my mind, body, and
spirit. I am so <u>thankful</u> !!*

Work in the nursing home in Leeds, Massachusetts was a
part of Stillpoint's contribution to the community and as students,
we also acquired diverse working experiences in these field
placements. At the nursing home, I witnessed human struggles
bound up with aging in our culture: the onset of Alzheimer's and
other diseases, compounded by loneliness and fear of the
unknown. I also saw extreme gentleness, grace, and courageous
acceptance of decline and death. The strength and wisdom of some
of the older people I met was inspiring. Even so, my own profound
struggles continued, unabated.

March 22, 1990
*Tonight Mary and I went to see My Left Foot. It
was an excellent movie, and very vividly recalled Ireland
and my childhood for me. The spark of human will and
the spirit to survive is what I must learn from this movie
and include in my life. Watching the scenes with
Christy's mother, I thought women are so amazing, so
powerful, so definitely the core of existence. The family
scenes tore at my heart: the brutal father, the endless
stream of babies, Christy's loneliness and isolation, the
yearning for love and the tenderness of a lover. The
hunger, the brilliance: the mind, the spirit, and the
body. My life shall not be transmuted; my desires are to
be risen above the ordinary.*

My Left Foot was about transcending, about how Christy
aspired to rise above his limitations of body, mind, and spirit.
Watching it quickened my heart and kindled a stronger flame of
spirit. It made me think about how to rise above simply the
struggle to survive, how to transcend my struggles, my suffering,
indeed, all struggles, and all sufferings. It recalled for me my
childhood suffering, fears, and abandonment—and at the same
time confronted me with my fears of being disabled, of ending up
in a wheelchair like my mother and my sister. In splitting off from
the fear, terror and powerlessness of my childhood state, I had

proceeded to create a super survivor persona.

Going to Nova Scotia, living out a back-to-the-land *healthy* and labour-intensive lifestyle had been a perfect environment in which to nurture the illusions of this strong-willed resourceful survival self. Deciding to take control of so many aspects of my physical survival, growing the food that we ate and then preserving it, preparing it, chopping and hauling the wood we used to keep warm, keeping a dairy cow—these things helped me to ward off the possible return of the feelings of that vulnerable, terrified, abandoned child I had been. Instead, I prided myself on my health and fitness, and I strove to be an example to myself, and others. And I was: I was admired and valued for these qualities of strength and self-provision. But as one friend put it, my "relentless resourcefulness" was above all an enormous defence mechanism.

The desire to be elevated above the ordinary is, of course, in part a wish to escape the ordinary or the mundane; as well, this wish emanates from the perception that there is or might be another reality, a larger and more inspired aspect of being towards which one might reach or strive. In his writings on the spiritual dimension of psychology, Assagioli described such an inspired aspect as the higher unconscious; it is that region of the psyche from which we receive our higher intuitions and aspirations, whether artistic, philosophical, scientific, or ethical imperatives, our urges to humanitarian and heroic action. Contrary to the Freudian view of the unconscious as the seat of all selfishness, anger, disappointment, and "base" passions, what Assagioli calls the higher unconscious greatly expands the domain of "hidden" human emotions and inspirations. The higher unconscious is the source within us of feelings such as altruistic love, of genius, and of the states of contemplation, illumination and ecstasy. In *My Left Foot*, Christy was very much in touch with this inspired higher unconscious as an artist, as well as in his struggles to transcend his physical limitations.

In my diary, I had continued my reflections upon the lessons that this movie held for my life:

To live ordinary life in a non-ordinary way. All around me are miracles of the enduring spirit—role models to last me a lifetime. What moods of pathos are with me now as I sit at this tiny desk looking at the photo of Irene and the photo of Mammy with us four youngest children. This 44th year has brought me to myself in a way that is changing the direction of my life. The inner work being done demands much change and focussed direction for my own learning, which will be different from the mind focus I have been in—returning me to my senses: my body, my emotions, and my intuitive spirit.

Ah yes, role models to last me a lifetime! My own mother, as I have mentioned, how her life had been constrained by her strict Catholic upbringing: the silencing of women, the suppression of her spirit through control, and the mandatory rules—thou shalt not use birth control; thou shalt not speak up against your husband's tyranny, let alone the tyranny of the church. Thou shalt not have freedom of thought and spirit, and if thou shouldst rebel, thou shalt suffer in sin and guilt for the rest of your days. As I have recounted, my mother did escape; she dared leave with her two youngest children, and, in her view, not only was she was punished by God with this dreadful arthritic disease, but she also had to watch her daughter be destroyed by the same disease for many long years. I know that my mother carried anger and hatred against my father with her to the grave. She never forgave him, nor, for that matter, did she ever forgive herself. As I see it, God did not need to punish her, for she punished herself. She never had any help to sort out her deep emotions of pain, guilt, loss, anger, rage and grief. What a human tragedy! She was the role model of a martyred Irish mother: how utterly she was destroyed. After the heroic deed of fleeing the country and the abusive relationship with my father, she could never get away from her sense of guilt and sin, her feeling that she had disobeyed God and all of the rules of the church patriarchy.

Likewise, my sister Irene did not get any help through those many torturous years in England. No one thought to suggest that she should see a therapist to work on the emotional material around her father's death, her refusal to see him, and, of course, the terror of her childhood, the terror of witnessing the violence, anger and abuse our father meted out to those around him.

As human beings, we can be crippled physically, but we can also be crippled emotionally and spiritually. The work I had begun at Stillpoint thus eventually pointed towards my need to seek psychological therapy, which I did in undertaking Psychosynthesis training. Because of Irene's financial support, perhaps because of her belated understanding of the importance of this kind of psychotherapeutic work, I was able to access the help I needed to do my deepest emotional healing work. At the same time, I was learning how to do this sort of work with others, but first, as our Psychosynthesis teacher insisted, we had to undertake a personal therapy, to work as hard as possible on our own healing. Thus the emphasis, particularly in the first year, was on doing such personal work, accompanied by readings and workshops and coursework. Of course, throughout the three years of my training, as an integral part of that training, I was in therapy with a Psychosynthesis therapist, striving in every way possible to fulfil the wisdom of the counsel that they who would be healers must first heal themselves. Thus it was that because of my sister Irene's support, I was able to undertake a process of psychological healing, as well as training in healing—a training which, in the end, helped us both.

But before all that happened, there were many rocky days. And nights.

> *Sunday, March 24, 1990*
>   *I called my sister today. She is having a very hard time; she can't breathe very well thanks to low white blood cell counts, which affect her breathing and cause her to have panic attacks. She has her care worker get her out of bed and take her to the hall door so that she can breathe the fresh air. She has been talking to her hospice nurse—planning in the event of her decline into death; they are discussing what interventions should or should not take place.*

Surprising as it might be now, at the time, I had not yet told

Irene about any of the pain and physical duress that I was going through. In fact, I did not tell her anything about my own suffering until I returned to Nova Scotia in June, despite the fact that during the whole of that spring I was closely connected to her through prayer and meditations. It was as if her suffering was my suffering then; I was finally able to understand the extent of her physical and emotional anguish over those many years that she struggled with her illness. I began to understand something about the abandonment that she must have felt when her husband left her, an abandonment which echoed the desertion she surely felt as a child when she listened, terrified, to the racket of our parents fighting, and our father's drunken rages. We shared that history, and now an illness. Later, I realized that I too feared that I would share another loss with Irene, that my partner would leave me to the ravages of my illness.

> *March 29, 1990*
> *Dream*
>   *Chris, the children, and I are getting on a spaceship to go to another planet. I am worried that we don't have enough food with us. There are other people on the voyage and I give them food, but there is not very much to go around....*

My dream late that March was quite prophetic, for it heralded a new way of life. I was indeed in the process of a change as great as that of moving to a new planet, a change that affected all of us drastically. Would we have enough food to sustain us in this new realm? Would I have what it took? Would I be able to provide what we needed? I set deadlines and made promises to myself, recording them in my diary.

> *March 31, 1990*
>   *The night before I give up all this tightness in my body, I am ready to let go and see Irene go to the arms of Mammy and Daddy and the beings of light. Tomorrow—April Fools Day—begins my release.*

Again and again I made up my mind that I would control my disease. If I were worth anything in this New Age cultural scene where I found myself, I would be able to cure myself, I thought. The illness that was in me would work out its course and leave, burn through my body, cleansing and purifying and preparing me, as a healer, to do my work. But things did not work out as I thought they would. Yes, I was purified in many respects, and I learned a great deal —and arthritis is still with me. I am still learning. Despite all my efforts on so many levels, my path includes my illness. My seeking after healing was crucial, but it did not bring what I thought it would. Today if you were to ask me what is healing, I would say healing is a condition of being at peace with who you are, nothing more and nothing less. It is not a state of physical perfection, of being super woman.

While at Stillpoint, however, I thought that if I was worthy (and worked hard enough) I could heal myself. I believed a version of what I now think of as New Age propaganda: You create your own reality; you can heal yourself—and if you do not, then whose fault is it? Another fine example of how easy it is for victims to fall into blaming themselves. Later I discovered a wonderful chapter entitled "Saints and Sinners" in Larry Dossey's inspiring book *Healing Words: The Power of Prayer and the Practice of Medicine*. Dossey cites numerous examples of very enlightened, self-realised people who suffered from numerous maladies and died of very common diseases, of which they obviously did not cure themselves. Often, their followers expected them to heal themselves, and were dumbfounded and uncomprehending of such a lesson in humility and fate. Dossey also offers as examples the tales of those sinners, the reprobates that we all know, who, despite eating all the "wrong" foods or smoking or drinking to excess, nevertheless manage to evade all the awful diseases associated with such "dangerous" living. Dossey's point, of course, is to challenge the self-righteousness of those of us who would control our risk factors, and everyone else's, those of us who believe we know the best way to live, and to die! For those of us who are into control, the state of affairs that Dossey describes is very tiresome. How dare there be no predictability in living and dying, no ultimate control in us over these processes! How dare we be left with only these things—struggle or acceptance? It has taken me a long time to learn these things. In truth, I am still learning, and I often forget, and fall back into old habits of wishing and thinking.

Even if control did not come to me, even if the physical healing I hoped for, and expected, would not arrive, interesting things were happening.

> *Sunday, April 1, 1990*
> *I talked to Irene and she said that the most extraordinary thing happened on Friday night. She woke, and could not go back to sleep. She panicked, then she thought of me and she felt my presence enter the room and kneel by the bed. She felt a great warmth in her heart area and, instantly, she fell asleep. I told her about my visualization in which she was going toward the light with Mammy and Daddy in a meadow of flowers. I explained that this was my visualization to try to enable me to let go of her (to allow her to die). I told her I loved her and that she was very special to me. Before we ended the phone call, she asked me to continue the visualization; she said she would call me in two weeks.*

Irene was, at the time, trying to let go and allow herself to die, but obviously, she was not ready. Perhaps she was still hanging on because of her children—although they were grown up, perhaps she was still hanging on because she had become so used to surviving. She had spent so many years concentrating on simply surviving that outwitting death was ingrained in her, a piece of her life force. It was hard for her to reverse the pattern of her survivor's life, to learn to let go. As it happened, she did not let go until five years later—on my last visit to her in March 1994. Four months later, in August, she finally died.

Seeing Irene struggle with so many medical treatments and the terrible side-effects of the drugs that she took for so many years certainly helped, initially, to turn me against the use of any drugs. Now, of course, I realize that if I had consulted doctors earlier and been willing to make use of available anti-arthritic drugs earlier, I would have experienced much less destruction in my knees, ankles, elbows, and shoulders. Rheumatoid arthritis is quite changeable; often it does not follow any clear pattern. In the realm of minor adjustments, it is thus very hard to know what helps and what does not, as the disease changes all the time. It is particularly difficult to know if diet, herbs, or other such treatments are working, because sometimes there is obvious relief and other times no change in one's state at all, whereas, when I took Chloroquine, the result was quick and obvious.

Today, after more than a decade of struggle with this illness and my own attitudes towards it, not to mention others' attitudes, I would argue that any rigidity, no matter how well meaning, is rigidity. In my refusal to use drugs in the first year of my illness, I was being rigid. Today, I would say to someone in the position that I found myself in 1990: Be smart, be flexible, use the best of both worlds. Be conscious of your diet, include vitamin supplements, avoid or limit alcohol and caffeine, but don't be afraid to use medication sensibly. Certainly, inform yourself of side-effects, but you must weigh the consequences of those side-effects of your medication against the progressive consequences of the disease. Where does the greatest risk of destruction lie? How will it affect your life? What you decide should be according to your informed choice, and not a pre-fixed stubborn notion of what 'should' be, for what *is* is often not what we imagine it 'should be.'

Tuesday, April 3, 1990
9:30 acupuncture. I told Margie about the visualization experience that Irene had, her feeling of me being present in her room. I also talked about how I am trying to let Irene go into the light with my mother and father in the meadow. She was very touched; she told me that she was treating me from an internal approach— from the earth, which is sympathy.

She felt that my pulses had improved since the last time I saw her. She burned moxa on my feet and put needles in my neck (sky pathways). I felt comforted for the first time in weeks—more gently accepting and grateful for life, for the lessons to be learned, for the work to do. The middle finger on my right hand was swollen. We looked at it and realized it was the heart meridian.

Throughout this whole period there was so much anguish in my heart, anguish that culminated in my heart opening to such a degree that afterwards I realized that a major shift had taken place.

> *Tuesday, April 10, 1990*
> *Acupuncture at 8:30: another experience of deep sadness welling up in me over Mammy—over leaving her when I was nineteen. I was remembering the fear I had of getting arthritis. Remembering her crying out in pain at night. I remember being impatient with her at times, and the terror of seeing both her and Irene so sick. I had to get away.*

There is no entry in my diary to detail the experience that I will now relate, but I know it happened around April of 1990, late one night, as I lay awake in agony and in the depths of despair. I was thinking about Mammy and Irene and feeling terrified that I was destined for a similar fate. I remember clearly the depths of despair that I felt when I really let down my guard. My diary is full of desperate attempts to fight off the experience of really allowing myself to get in touch with the pain and the grief, the anger and the rage that I was experiencing regarding the people and events in my life, in particular, my feelings about my sister, my mother, and my childhood. I felt the return of my childhood terror, faced as I was with anguish and despair at how thoroughly everything I had planned had fallen apart. What happened on that night would, in the end, change my life. It set me on a new path: that of a consciously self-actualizing being. As I lay on my bed, unable to move, in an agony of physical and emotional pain, filled with despair and a deep sense of failure, I experienced an incredible loss of hope. I felt terror in my heart. I was convinced that I had fallen into an abyss from which I would never emerge. This utterly despairing part of me rarely wrote in the diary. Everything in the world seemed dark, and then, at that awful moment, from the depths of the abyss, just when I had abandoned all hope—an incredible feeling came over me, a feeling of the opening of my heart. I was surrounded by light and filled with a feeling of extraordinary bliss. There, all around me was so much love and joy—indescribable joy, which lasted several hours. The next day, something of the experience stayed with me. I found that I looked on those around me with far more compassion and acceptance. Suddenly, I found it far easier to accept unconditionally the people whom I felt posed some difficulty in and to my life. I was far less embattled, and I found myself crying with gladness, an over-brimming of beauty and joy. Such a softening of my heart took me by surprise; I felt an enormous tenderness for others.

A close friend who came to visit me that following day found me ecstatic— brimming over with love and tenderness. I was easily moved to tears by any act of kindness. Her daughter had sent me a card with a lovely childish greeting and it touched me deeply.

You may well ask, what new development was at hand here? How could the experience of profound despair give way to an experience of bliss? In this new state, I felt slowed down, everything was slowed down, which made me realize how thoroughly my usual busy activities destroyed any sense of peace that I might have; the drive of my everyday life was the opposite of the blissful state I was in, where everything was more relaxed, effortless, easier, calmer. I recalled the feelings I had had on acid: how beautiful the world seemed, and too, how *still* I became. With this new state came a new challenge never afforded by drug-induced bliss: how might one get to a point somewhere in between driveness and stillness? How might I let go of my compulsive activity, and find a gentler, more peaceful pace?

For several days, the feeling of beatific calm stayed with me, and I was left with the knowledge that something new and very powerful had entered my life. Without the aid of hallucinatory drugs, I had experienced a state of consciousness quite different from my normal reality. This was a state, I would learn, which Assagioli had described as the "true source and essence of being." In other words, I had had a mystical or peak experience, and it left me with a longing to know and to experience such states again. I began to see that I needed to bring such spiritual qualities of peace and calm, compassion, and acceptance into my daily life. If this was the true source and essence of being, I wanted more of it in my life! Unfortunately, however, such transcendental experiences are not things that one may turn on at will. Still it awakened me to life in a way that I had not experienced before; it changed my world view. From that moment on, I knew that my goal was to try to bring this potential source and essence of being into every aspect of my life. I had been called: my mystical experience confirmed for me the spiritual as my true nature, and it set me on a rich and fruitful spiritual quest that has not ended to this day.

> *Friday, April 13, 1990*
> *Good Friday—acupuncture at 11am. Margie is trying the amazing "Pubescent Angelica Mulberry Mistletoe Soup" for my sore and stiffened joints. We had a good session: needles at the base of my head, knees, feet, ankles, hands, wrists, and on the meridian lines. Saturday I cleaned her office and painted all afternoon. It felt wonderful to feel so good and to do some work. Friday I went to Boyden for the crystals. He had Joan do some friction on trigger points for the adrenals.*

Up to that point, the program had included dieting, fasting, acupuncture, Chinese herbs, chiropractic treatments, laying crystals in disks under my body, meditation, yoga, vitamin supplements, prayer, affirmations, consulting tarot cards, and recording my dreams. I wanted desperately to get well; I thought that all I had to do was to find the right thing for me. I was sure that if, out of all these disciplines I was trying, I could find it, then I would get well. Ah! Alas! if only life were so simple.

> *Easter Sunday morning*
> *Raining heavy, mild. I called home at 9 o'clock and talked to everyone. I am missing them so much. I am creating positive thoughts to counteract the negative*

aspects of this disease. I realize I have been separated from myself through fear and lack of self-love. I must remember to keep the message and memory of this illness in my heart and mind so that I can use the knowledge gained to help others.

What motivated me to take as my mission helping others for all of those years? Was it the only reason for being, the only activity that I felt was justified? When I think about it now, I realize that I gained a lot of self-worth through helping others. I felt that I was accepted and valued because of my work in the battered women's shelter or in feeding or fighting for the rights of others. What I could offer was my strength, my capacity to care for those less well off than I. This sense was, in part, what sent me to Stillpoint for training in massage and holistic healing. In my activities over the years, I had cared for many others; I strove to be deeply compassionate, and I maintained a fierce and fighting sense of justice. But despite my abilities to look after others, I neglected and abandoned my self. I had contempt for the so-called "weaker" parts of my self, my "lost self." I had very little patience or compassion for her feelings, her terror, and her powerlessness. I had to be the one who was in control all of the time; I must be the one who had that relentless resourcefulness; I prided myself on my ability to help others; there was no room in my vision of myself for one who, herself, might be in need.

Suddenly, however, I was in a position where I could no longer actively help others; in fact, I *had* to accept help from others. How difficult that was! And it became even more difficult when I returned home to Nova Scotia in a much-diminished physical state. How could I make the adjustment to a different way of life? Relying as I did on my work of helping others for my sense of self-worth, what was I to do? I had a hard time believing that I was worthy of love and acceptance just as I was. Thus I embarked on a very important learning process, and it took some time for me to absorb the necessary lessons at a deep level. In fact, I am still working at them.

Here I am, more than a decade later, still coping with this chronic persistent disease. There is no doubt that it has taught me a great deal that I can use to help others, but reaching out to others has a different meaning now than it once did. I've come to realize that both illness and healing are far more complex than I ever imagined they would be. Usually when someone falls seriously ill, whether physically or psychically, there is no simple answer, no magic bullet, no easy cure. Each person is different and every disease behaves differently in each person. Modes of treatment that work for one person may not work for another. And in the process of any grave illness, you are confronted with all sorts of emotional challenges: how do you work with your anger, pain, grief, and denial; how do you accept and learn from your feelings, so that they may serve rather than hinder your healing? In any long-term or chronic illness, any experience of decline, there is also the struggle to understand that healing may not mean that one will be cured of the disease, but rather that you come to a means of living with it. This is often a very hard lesson— especially for people like me who have spent many years of their lives focused on (self) control.

At school, everyone was aware of the struggles I was going through. My pathology teacher asked me if I had considered getting tested for Lymes disease. I looked up the symptoms of Lymes disease in my textbooks and found that they included arthritic-type pains in the joints; I was especially interested to read that these pains often felt as if they migrated from one joint to the other in the body. I decided getting tested was worth a try. Who knows? Maybe a cure was just around the corner! Maybe I was looking for the right treatment, without knowing the name of the disease.

Tuesday, April 17, 1990

I met with my acupuncturist and told her about my decision to be tested for Lymes disease. Amy gave me the lab form to get the test done. I will know in a week.

Wednesday, April 25, 1990
Margie called today to say the test was positive,
which blew me away. I have tested positive for Lymes
disease! Astonishing! I keep thinking that it can't be
the right test. The diagnosis has to be more complex
than a simple antibody test will show. Mary is calling to
get me an appointment with a Lymes disease specialist.
I hope I can get to see him soon. If this is true, I guess I
will be put on a mega dose of antibiotics....

As it turned out, of course, I did not have Lymes disease. Too bad —in a way! If it had been the cause of so much of my pain, I could have taken lots of antibiotics and, hopefully, they would have killed it off. No more pain, no more destruction! But that was not to be. Instead, in the course of my visit to the specialist, I was tested for rheumatoid arthritis and that test came back positive. How depressing that was! I remember standing in the doctor's office when he said, "It is more likely that you have rheumatoid arthritis than Lymes disease. I think you should have a blood test and find out for sure, so that you can start treatment to get these symptoms under control." These words rang like a death knell in my ears; when the test returned positive I was stunned. For several months, in fact, I could not admit that it was true: I was suffering from rheumatoid arthritis. Consequently, I delayed getting medical help, which meant that I experienced even greater destruction in my knees than necessary. Stubbornly, I was still convinced that I did not need to take any pharmaceutical drugs; I felt that I could heal myself by using more natural methods. I continued to try out as many healing systems as I could find.

Under duress of all kinds, I graduated from massage school and closed a chapter of my life that had had a shattering impact on me. In less than a year, I had undergone quite a change. Life would never be the same again. It took me several weeks after I returned to Nova Scotia to work up the courage to write and tell my sister that I too had rheumatoid arthritis. I wrote to her rather than called because I had to think about how I would explain why it took me so long to tell her. As I expected, upon receiving my news, she was very shocked and very upset. In fact, she told me later, she was extremely angry, perhaps because my affliction with the illness enabled her, in a way that her own experience did not, to get in touch with her own deep anger at what damage the disease wreaked.

I did not know what to say or how to respond to the fear and anger that she had that I, her little sister, appeared not to have escaped her hard fate. My whole family in England were very shocked and very concerned; having seen so much pain and destruction at the hands of this disease, they feared the worst. All of these family emotions made me even more frightened. I did not want to go out and see people and I could not bear to have them see me as I was, barely able to walk. I did not want to talk about what was wrong or how I was feeling. My children and my partner had a very difficult time. My daughter became very angry with me; she argued that this never would have happened if I had stayed at home with her. We were all caught in a swirl of hurt, pain, and anger, and there were no easy solutions.

My family doctor tried to encourage me to take Chloroquine, an anti-malarial drug, which seemed to work well to control arthritis. I refused to take it. I did agree to take a less powerful non-steroidal anti-inflammatory, which helped for a while but could not keep my high inflammatory rate under control. I was barely coping; I continued to lose weight, and I was in terrible pain. I was also working part-time doing research. Now when I think about it, I am amazed that I managed to do anything at all, given the horrendous pain I was often in. Finally, a year or more after my diagnosis I went down to Halifax to see a rheumatologist. He was an older, kindly, Welsh man. He took one look at me and took over; he insisted that I be admitted to the hospital immediately, for at least two weeks. He got me started on Chloroquine, injected both my knees with Cortisone, and gave me a serious talking to about how far I had let myself go. I was down to 105 pounds from an original weight of 130 pounds. He was absolutely right, of course; in my ferocity concerning the control of my body, things had gotten totally out of control.

It was such a relief to let go, to rest, to let others take care of me. I was so deeply exhausted and the pain had taken such a toll on me that I was happy to let others fuss over me. The survivor part of me had battled on for so long; I had been convinced that to give in, to give up, was a sign of weakness. But now I was pushed against the wall and had to surrender. In truth, I was delivered.

CHAPTER III

The Heroic Response

Relinquish struggle, let go, stop the battle for control, and accept what is! I had tried so hard to control this illness, to control my response to it, and my recovery. I had decided that I would recover by a certain time and by certain methods only. From the onset of my illness, this struggle ensued, and over the course of the next decade, in a process that is still ongoing, I learned a great deal about surrender and acceptance. Like peeling the proverbial onion, I would get through one layer of resistance only to be confronted by another.

When I examine the experiences I have described during the year at Stillpoint, several things stand out for me regarding my beliefs:

> * I saw my illness as a failure on my part.
> * I believed I had to be healthy and fit all of the time.
> * I was convinced that I had to heal myself.
> * I did not allow for the part that my emotions, of fear, terror, and powerlessness, might play in my well-being.
> * If illness stemmed from the spirit as I thought it

did, I concluded that I must be spiritually deficient if I could not heal myself.

* I believed that if I was good enough, I would get well.

* I refused conventional medicine; it didn't know anything about me that I couldn't discover myself.

* Grief and guilt were profound aspects of my suffering; as I developed the same illness that overtook my mother and sister, the pain and guilt that I felt at having abandoned them when they became ill emerged.

* Illness involved confronting the twin monsters of terror and abandonment.

* I believed that for it to be justified, I must find meaning in my illness.

Again and again, as the illness began its work on me, I fell prey to what I would call 'the heroic response'— I would not allow myself any weakness. The survivor part of me would take over, and look after everything. In this way, I protected myself from my most profound and terrifying senses of failure.

My sense of failure and my belief that I had to be fit all the time were two parts of the same whole. Like many others in our culture, I saw illness as failure, or perhaps even punishment for wrongdoing or selfishness. I could not understand that illness was as much a part of the fabric of life as birth or death. In this sense, I was not different from nearly everyone else I knew: we all believed that the very best way to live was to try to avoid pain and suffering, to try to be as comfortable as we could be. But perhaps comfort is not the end that we imagine that it is, particularly a comfort achieved thanks to a denial of our vulnerabilities, our fragilities, our very real proximity, as soon as we are alive, to death.

My belief that I had to heal myself—'I created this illness; I had to heal it'— had been picked up through my reading of New Age literature. Eventually, after a good deal of self-torture, I let go of the notion I had to heal myself. Indeed, I stopped understanding "healing" as something that meant "getting rid of the arthritis," for arthritis continued to be my constant companion. And even if illness somehow stemmed from the spirit, I came to believe I was not spiritually deficient because I was ill and could not cure myself. Eventually, I would come to realize that wholeness existed in me even in the height of my illness: my essence, my essential spirit, was and is always luminously present. The great difficulty was coming to see and to celebrate this fact.

For a long long while, I fought desperately to ward off pain, suffering and illness, doing all sorts of mental and spiritual gymnastics. My life was filled up with healing practices, and I continued to become less and less well. Down deep, as I performed all of those fasts and purifications and exercises, I held on to the belief that if I was good enough, if I did my dietary or planetary calisthenics well enough, I would get better. It took a long time for me to see that such beliefs were a return to the world of my Catholic childhood: the fear of constant and unintentional sin against which I had to be on my guard, augmented, of course, by a good deal of magical thinking. I tried my best to be selfless in my every action, to be filled with goodness and well wishing for others, but I had to let that bit of magic go too. Despite having the best of intentions for everyone, I had yet to find the best of intentions for myself— my life, my freedom, and my potential self.

It is very hard for Christians who are raised with a strong sense of original sin, the tale of the fall into knowledge, which is also the fall into evil, and the impossibility of redemption without divine intervention, to come to accept the richness and depth of their basic goodness, to believe that they too possess a divine nature. Exposure to some of the beliefs of Buddhism helped me to overcome my sense of my fundamental sinfulness and allowed me to begin to hope again. It was a challenge to believe that I was good, worthy, and sacred—perhaps coming to grips with such truth is the ultimate challenge for all of us. In time, my training in Psychosynthesis would help to underscore even more the importance of such a generous belief in my higher self and the worthiness of my spiritual nature.

When I first came home from Stillpoint, I read an article by

Ken Wilber that asked, "Do we create our own illness?" Written with the intent of examining New Age beliefs around illness and healing, Wilber's article challenged my thinking. Later, he produced a book with his wife Treya about her struggle with terminal cancer. Called *Grace and Grit,* their book is a moving and insightful exploration of many of the major questions a person confronts in facing illness and death. As they discuss, one of the key messages in popular New Age approaches to health and wellness is that the ideal is optimum physical health—and if we are tuned in on a properly calibrated spiritual and emotional energy system, in a perfect mind and body connection, then we can, (and should be able to) achieve optimum health. What happens in such a system, however, when catastrophic accident or terminal illness strikes? What resources does it offer? Not very many. In such a system, those who do not fit the image of the vibrant, glowing, fit, able body are rendered silent, shamed, marginal, invisible, unacceptable. Sinners, who deserve only to be cast out as so many broken shards or husks. In the end then, as the Wilbers argue, when put to the test, much of the promise and apparent generosity of certain New Age views breaks down, and the harshness and inhumanity of a view of humanity which does not see illness as a part of life, rather than its opposite, shows through.

Rachel Naomi Remen adds fuel to such a critique in her article "Imagery and the Search for Healing." In this essay, she challenges readers with the assumption that illness is one of the conditions that evokes wholeness or leads to wholeness. A medical doctor who has worked extensively with cancer patients, Rachel Naomi Remen is also a trained psychosynthesis practitioner. She suggests that far more important to healing than an abstract idea of wellness is a perspective that allows both healer and patient to understand that "not everything can be fixed, not everything that appears to need fixing is broken." In this manner, as a doctor, she does what she can, medically speaking, to promote physical health; she also supports those spiritual and psychical processes within us, whether we are physically well or not, which move us to greater wholeness.

We may not know what meanings are evoked by our

illnesses or misfortunes. Many of us, upon falling ill, search desperately for meaning to make sense of what has happened to us. We witness quite extraordinary examples of such struggles after meaning in the lives of people like Victor Frankl, who, in his book *Man's Search for Meaning* wrote about his experiences in a concentration camp during World War II. It seems that most of us want to believe that there is some plan, that there are reasons for the various challenges we encounter, and that we are, each and every one of us, special. Most of us, at one point or another, come around to the sense that life is precious, and that each of our lives is part of something greater, something that we might call a divine plan.

Our everyday lives in the world lead us away from such a spiritual sensibility because our lives are, for the most part, outer-directed. For most of us, our primary goals are what I would call 'survivor goals.' We aim to get an education, to earn a living, to raise a family, and our priorities are to make money and be happy, to seek after truth—in that order. Indeed, you may do everything on your list of goals to be achieved and still long for something more. What will it take for you to seek what you long for? Often enough, when our lives are thoroughly outer-directed, it takes a crisis to bring us to some sort of inner reflection. We become aware of our inner landscape, and our quest for a life beyond 'survival mode' begins.

If I had been healed, if I had gone into remission or found a drug that cured my illness, doubtless I would have returned to living my life in the speedy outer-directed fashion that I had pursued before my illness. Instead, coming as it did, without a cure, my illness pushed me to examine my life, to attend to my emotional and spiritual health. I began to try to live my life more authentically, which is also to say, more fully than I ever did when I was in the very "bloom" of physical health. When I talked to other people who struggled with illness, many of them said that they too were pushed to find their real selves, their true feelings, to take an honest look at their relationships, sometimes to take the risk of getting out of a job they hated or a relationship that was damaging. Often, they said, they had to confront dysfunctional behaviours that were holding them back from fully living their lives. Illness, then, can be an important and active incentive to growth!

In the first five years of my illness, the greatest challenge that I faced was to try to find meaning and forward motion *in* my illness and not simply *despite* it. As I see it now, my life needed to change —I needed to slow down and to work on my own very personal recovery from early childhood wounds and their consequent effects on my life. I also needed to change or re-adjust certain behavioral patterns, in order to free up my energies to live my life more authentically. Meanwhile, all around me the race was on for me to get well. In a culture bent on seeing good health or lack of illness as the norm, there was tremendous pressure to shape up, to get better, to get over it. In such a whirl, Kat Duff's little book *The Alchemy of Illness* was inspirational. There, she argued that

> *the sense of diminishment we so often experience in the grasp of the unknowable, the face of the incurable, probably has something to offer us from a spiritual perspective, but in the secular world of twentieth century America, it is without meaning and so intolerable.*

Her book helped me to see that in this culture, the first commandment of illness is to get well, and if we don't, there is hell to pay. I began to try to understand why, rather than berating myself for not "shaping up" properly.

It became evident to me that most of us in this technologically fixed West are terrified of aging and change. The heroic qualities most valued in our culture are youth, activity, productivity, independence, strength, confidence and optimism. Health becomes an impossible ideal. Faced with a silver screen idol and ideal, utter plastic perfection, we have come to equate that perfection with what is normal. In fact, deviation from that norm is not only the rule, but also what is far more interesting! These "imperfections" and deviations shape our characters and identify our uniqueness. Growing up in Ireland as a child, where there was little money for dental work and orthodontists were not an option, if you had buck teeth, then that's what you had, no big deal. It was part of your character, part of who you were. Flat feet, big noses, flat chests, warts, moles, lameness: these were all distinguishing features, not aspects to be erased by plastic surgery or other orthopedics.

Today, in this culture, we are expected to conform to standards of normality, of great health. And even if the majority of us do not, as individuals, we struggle with deep senses of failure. Such ruin of self-worth has only been compounded by the cheery messages of many New Age helpers bent on whipping us into shape.

Illness is not the great evil, the great failure. Very often, it can push us to work with our deepest beliefs about ourselves. Falling ill may move us to greater levels of healing and wholeness, greater levels of introspection and self- and other-understanding. We may be forced, through the circumstances of chronic illness, to work with profound levels of trust and belief in our own basic goodness and wholeness. Gratitude for what we have, and the ability to see the richness of our lives in their many dimensions, is often the gift we gain from such circumstances. We also learn that living with limitation is very normal and very human, and that we can embrace this humanness in ourselves.

LEARNINGS AND MEDITATIONS

ACCEPTANCE – LETING GO THE BATTLE FOR CONTROL

Learnings
Meditations

How can we know the right time for surrender and acceptance?
We may battle long and hard to control a situation that is beyond
our control. We may launch a battle of denial and resistance
against an unwanted state of being or illness. All the feelings of
failure, terror and powerlessness that these situations bring up in
us must be accepted and experienced instead of running from them.
Acceptance is surrendering to them. At first we may see this as a
sign of weakness but actually it is an act of courage to allow
ourself to experience the suffering. Acceptance can then be a form
of power, a life affirming choice instead of resistance and
resentment. With acceptance we can move foreword with grace and
dignity, acknowledging the gifts and teachings in the situation
which enriches our lives.

Meditation on Acceptance

Adapted from Ferucci's What We May Be

Seated comfortably, bring your attention inside, connect with your breath, rest in your breathing. Become aware of a quiet space within. Breathe and relax. Now allow yourself to reflect on what is happening in your life right now – all of the experiences good or not so good. Allow yourself to be open and curious. Take a few moments and let that go. Now allow yourself to think about something in your life for which you are truly grateful – a friend, a loved one, your child, the beauty of nature – whatever. Allow it to be present – vivid and alive in your imagination – appreciate it – think of what it gives you and what you learn from it.

Now think of somebody or something you would like to avoid in your life. Imagine it as vividly as you can and watch closely any reactions that arise in you. Just observe your habitual strategies of non-acceptance in your body, mind and feelings – stay with that for a time.

Now let that go and imagine that life is communicating with you in a code language made up of situations and events. What is the message in this situation or event? What can it teach you to enrich your life?

Now return to the situation or event you felt grateful for. Imagine it vividly and be fully aware of your acceptance, notice how that is in your body, mind and feelings. Note the lightness and joy. Now switchback to the unpleasant situation bringing with you the accepting attitude. Realize that the same universe that produced what was pleasant also produced what was unpleasant and assume if you feel ready an attitude of conscious deliberate acceptance.

Breathe and rest.

CHAPTER IV

Ritual

Healing comes not only from inside of us but also through community; very often it is evoked through ritual. Of course, rituals can also be solitary. Often, however, they have a particular power and meaning when they involve a group. When I first came back to Nova Scotia after my difficult year at Stillpoint, my first wish and deepest longing was to make my way to the ocean. In particular, I wanted to go to a very familiar and very beautiful beach, a beach that, over the years, had been a major meeting place for a small group of my women friends.

Four years earlier, I had celebrated my fortieth birthday with this group of women on that beach. I remember it was an exquisite evening: the sun dropping like a fire into the ocean, the clouds ablaze with crimson light. Someone spread a blanket on the sand and covered it with a white lace tablecloth, crystal wine glasses, champagne, and all sorts of delicious foods. We ate well, and then, at last, the cake was produced. It was magnificent, gorgeous, an excess of chocolate, baked by a dear friend who knew my tastes well. Not content to have baked a delicious and wonderful chocolate cake and frosted it with rich chocolate icing, my friend had taken hours to shape chocolate petals by hand, which she then pressed into the cake, interspersed with the hot pink mallow flowers that bloom everywhere in the late summer. The whole effect was just as she—and I—wished: a delight to the eye and a sensation to the palate.

This group of friends had gathered to celebrate my age, to honour forty years, to ritualise the passage of time in my life. Together, they reminded me of my gifts—of the power of self-choice, and of the richness and beauty of my womanhood, my selfhood. For me, around me, I felt that this sacred circle of women carried the continuity of life: here was the life-giving lineage of women, the capacity for childbearing, for forever creating life anew in our art and craft. This was a caring, inspiring female community which brought together the all too often separate spheres of hearth, home and the public realm. Together we bore witness to destruction, abuse, and neglect, which we addressed by consciousness-raising, and together we conspired to renew, redress, replenish, and restore one another and the world around us. Together, we celebrated the Goddess in our image; we re-imagined ourselves and our bodies. Inspired by images of the Goddess and the history of her influence and power, we reclaimed our bodies from the destructions our lives and patriarchal culture had wreaked on our self-respect; we came to see our own flesh, too, as divine, as sacred. Honouring ourselves, together we also honoured every other life force: earth, sky, flower and seed, river and spring, ocean wave, bird and beast.

Over the years then we came together to rediscover the beauty within ourselves, within each other. We were humbled and exalted by the beauty in us and around us. Over the years, we had used this beach, this sacred space, as a gathering place to remember who we were. Here we would gather to remind ourselves and each other of our sacredness, and to mark the changing seasons, of the years, and of our lives. In this circle, we grieved our losses: the dying, the pain and suffering of life. Together, we celebrated the joy and beauty of living, the birthing, the work accomplished, the battles won and lost. We consulted the oracle with Tarot and Rune stones. We built altars—stone circles decorated with flowering sea pea plants, shells, fruit, and candles set in the sand around the hearth of our fire.

On summer solstice, we prayed to Yemaya, the ocean goddess, and pushed wishing boats, made of leaves, out to sea. Every year on June 21st in Nova Scotia, we waded into the icy water. We set red candles in the sand in the form of a semicircle at the edge of the ocean. There was the blue velvet darkness of the sky, the murmur of the waves on the beach, the candlelight flickering on the shore, the presence of women who had sustained and supported each other's growth. This is what I remember year after year: the beauty of our bodies, the strength of our limbs, our contagious laughter and tears. Together we wove a human tapestry, which in its fabric revealed every sort of light, dark shadow and chaos. Together we charted and survived the gaping abysses, the pinnacles and plateaus of movements gained, of successes, losses, and completions.

Over the course of twenty years, many women had come and gone from this group, weaving in and out as they moved to new places in the world and in their lives. At least five or six of us remained constant, however, always there to carry the flame of the circle of sisters. But everyone, no matter how far-flung from our Nova Scotia shore, remained present in our hearts.

Thus it was that in my state of pain, suffering, and bewilderment, I was drawn, within the circle of the group, to the healing shores and healing water of our sacred place. And because I could barely walk, the members of the group bore me up; they helped me to make my way through the deep sand to our appointed spot. I sat on a folding chair, elevated above the group, for I could no longer sit on the ground. And when it got cold I became so stiff that I could hardly move, despite being tucked all around with blankets. Nevertheless, I was glad to be there. I looked around the circle and felt the strength of these good friends all around me. With them I knew that I was loved and valued, just as I was at any given moment in any given state. Even when my pain and despair leaked through and tinged my joy and delight.

For as long as I can remember, these rituals have sustained me. It is no accident, I am sure, that I sought out the company of my circle of friends when I felt most deeply lost. All my life, my instinct had been very strongly in pursuit of beauty. As a child, when my home environment became violent, chaotic and restrictive, I had created a sacred space in response: setting up an altar in my bedroom to Mary, the Queen of Heaven. Then, particularly in May, the month of Mary, I would gather wildflowers, fill jam pots with them, and set them on my altar. Rambling through the countryside in pursuit of primroses, daffodils, violets, daisies, cowslips, snowdrops, each in its season, had been my time of greatest freedom and joy. And, of course, in my childhood home in rural southern Ireland, I inhabited a land of ruined castles, sacred wells, and mystical sites. Tales attached to the landscape were all around me. One of the most important sites for me was Newbury Pond, the place where the River Boyne rose. Not only was it a lovely place, but the rising of this fabled river featured prominently in the myths of Ireland, for it was from the River Boyne that Fionn MacCumhaill had pulled the salmon of knowledge. As I recall it, the river's source was a magical place: water sprang from a rock surrounded by moss, gushing clear and rippling out through the pond, and flowed onward to form the great river. Newbury Pond was part of an estate built by landed English gentry, a fact which made it necessary for me to climb the ivy covered wall which edged the estate in order to make my way to the edge of the pond. Beauty and secrecy were thus bound together for me. How much I loved the stillness and beauty there!

"I come from haunts of coot and heron." Yes, indeed, I do come from the haunts of the great blue heron, where there were also magnificent trees, waters dappled by lily pads, fish jumping in the pools and, in the spring, the most magnificent carpets of wild daffodils, thickly clustered under giant elms in the nearby meadow. Such beauty lifted me up, beyond the mundane, to touch the Divine. Here, in this untouched pristine world, I could lose myself— and all of the sorrows and worries of my everyday child's life. Here I was free. Here I somehow felt that there was meaning, a plan beyond human origin or imagination.

It took many years—until my Psychosynthesis training— before I was able to begin to do the work necessary to heal the wounds of my childhood. Like so many others who are traumatized or abused at a young age, I had split myself off from the pain and suffering in me and around me. In order to survive, I created various controlling mechanisms to block out the memory of the pain and terror of my childhood. Being alone in nature was a solace and an escape; it had been so my entire life. As it turned out, being able to be out in the natural world and to take pleasure in it, not only by myself but also with others was also an important route to my recovery.

I remember being very struck when I first read the preface to Alice Miller's poignant book *The Drama of the Gifted Child*, in which she states that

> *We live in a culture that encourages us not to take our own suffering seriously, but rather to make light of it or even to laugh about it. What is more, this attitude is regarded as a virtue, and many people, of whom I used to be one, are proud of their lack of sensitivity toward their own fate, and particularly toward their fate as a child.*

Like so many others, I had learned to dismiss and minimize my pain; thus, at first, I treated my pain by denying my needs and feelings, a move that simply perpetuated the cycle within which I was trapped.

In childhood, beauty and the creation of sacred spaces had been very important for my survival. The rituals in which I set up altars were done alone. In later years, inspired by my circle of women friends, I was again drawn to ritual expressions and activities, to chanting, dancing, and drumming. Instinctively, somehow, I seemed to know that ritual was an important and healing force in my life. At first, what was most important was the experience of becoming one with the group and transcending the small self, becoming part of the flow around me. When I watched the sunset over the ocean, I became the sunset and the waves lapping the shore. I became my sister; her pain was my pain. Her joy was my joy. In our circle, we held among us the strengths and the frailties of all humans. We reminded each other that we were both human and Divine. In our hours of deepest despair, we held each other up.

Life is suffering, said the Buddha. But when I first came back from Stillpoint, I was having a very hard time with so much suffering. I wanted no part of it. I wanted to go back to being "normal," whatever that was. I wanted to be healed of this awful physical affliction. I wanted to bound back into my old and busy, active life again.

Alas! If only life were so simple! Would a return to the way things had been have been the best thing for me? Today, I am not sure. If I had been healed of my affliction so speedily, I doubt that I would have heard let alone retained the message of my illness, the news that you live in a body, you have a mind and experience emotions, you live out everyday dramas—but the fullness of life consists of so much more than any of these things in isolation! We are spiritual beings, made manifest in a physical body. I had to come to understand that my illness was my spiritual practice. Every day, my struggles with my body reminded me of the limits of my obsessions with my body; every day I learned anew that I was and am more than simply the sum of my body. This daily lesson became my strength and inspiration. I had to learn to dis-identify—a move that is not the same as disassocia-tion!— from my body with all of its aches and pains. I had to develop the sense that my *true self* included but was more than this poor, fragile body, unique and wonderful as it was.

Our bodies can be sources of wonder and delight, but they can also at times become prison houses of torture and pain. In 1990, I began to learn about the latter, and I struggled fiercely. My response was to reject and recoil from the pain and deformity that afflicted me, to reject and recoil from myself. Rheumatoid arthritis brings twisted limbs, swollen and crooked hands and feet, and a stiffened gait—when you can still move around at all. It was all so unfair! It made me terribly angry, but beneath my anger there was so much grief and loss that I could not begin to count it.

My friends stayed with me; the faithfulness and support of that close circle of women was important, indeed crucial, to me. But I also had work to do that only I could do alone. There were inner demons to be conquered, or, more precisely, to be befriended. In the past I had tried to conquer the demons and subdue them, to exorcise and annihilate them. The practice of Psychosynthesis taught me to befriend them instead. Borne up by the love of others, I struggled with this lonesome inner work and my spirit was revealed to me. As I slowly came to recognize, my spirit was burnished ever brighter with the workings of my pain. At first, I simply experienced brief glimpses of it in the darkness, reminders that I was still whole, despite my sufferings, perhaps even more so because of them.

Slowly, I dropped the notion that the only acceptable way to be healthy was to be sound in limb and glowing in that vibrant, perfectible, functioning body of idealized *normal* standards. I had to break free of the jail of that mentality, and as I did, my moods flew up and down. Some days I experienced despair, other days self-pity or self-loathing. On still other days, I felt calm, peaceful, and accepting, and occasionally I even experienced delight and joy to be alive in the world.

But always, whenever doubt assailed me, I returned to the quiet power and dignity of my rituals of sacredness, whether alone, or together in the group. These rituals offered support and meaning to this critical period of change in my life, as they had done in the past. They anchored me, and gave me the occasion formally to invoke the blessings of the Goddess in my time of crisis, danger, and opportunity. They served me well, and continue to be very rich and powerful aspects of my life.

LEARNINGS AND MEDITATIONS

RITUAL

Learnings
Meditations

Healing through ritual, beauty and the aesthetic sense. Assagioli presented beauty as one of the most powerful and regenerative healing influences in our lives. He encouraged his students to seek out beauty and surround themselves with it – what ever inspires us with delight and uplifts our heart and spirit – art, nature, music, dance…. Beauty lifts us into expansive awareness, it portends a promise of fulfillment and possibility or maybe a remembrance of lost bliss – a sense of longing for the Divine. When we combine beauty and ritual we can be uplifted and restored to the realm of unlimited possibility.

Meditation on Ritual and Beauty
To evoke the highest realm of possibility.

Seated comfortably, bring your attention inside, connect with your breath, rest in your breathing. Become aware of a quiet space within you. Breathe and relax.

Now if you are willing find yourself walking in nature in some very beautiful place with special meaning to you. Some place where you feel safe and surrounded by beauty. It may be a beach or near a lake or waterfall. It may be in a beautiful building or temple – whatever it is feel free to include aspects of beauty that are particularly uplifting to you. As you enter this space be aware that this is a very sacred place in which you can conduct a ritual to celebrate your unique beauty and sacredness.

You may wish to have certain objects in this sacred space – stones, shells, flowers, an eagle feather. Arrange this space as simply or elaborately as you wish. When you feel satisfied gaze around you and take in the beauty of this ritual space. In the center of your space imagine a table or rock on which a small simple bowl containing water rests. This water represents the primordial waters from whence you came and will be used in a ritual self-blessing. You may wish to bear witness and mark a change, new beginning or honour your power wisdom and potential. As you lift the bowl of water and sprinkle drops on your forehead, heart and stomach repeat if you will: I who carry the light of the world, the spark of the Divine bless my body, mind and feelings that they may be illumined as they illuminate my life. May I live in respect and reverence of all that is in me – all those around me, respect the divine that flows through me and all the universe. May I awake to my power and my gifts, my beauty. The love and beauty within, may I know and experience my boundless possibility and potential. Bless myself and blessed be.

Hold that sacred ritual space as long as you need and know that you can return whenever you wish.

Breathe and rest.

CHAPTER V

Psychosynthesis: The Soul's Path

In the summer of 1992, I enrolled in a weeklong workshop called The Seven Paths to the Soul. I had gone through an incredible amount of pain and suffering on many levels in the two years since my diagnosis. My path had often led me through very rough terrain; as I now see, I was stumbling about in search of my Dharma, my soul's purpose. Again and again I returned to a feeling of great longing, an urge to seek or to uncover my destiny, my lifework and goal in this lifetime. What was the meaning of my life? What would it be?

I remember one afternoon, when I'd driven to my partner's workplace to pick him up. As I waited, I read the program of workshops offered in the coming year at the Atlantic Christian Training Center (ACTC), a beautiful retreat center on the water near Tatamagouche, Nova Scotia. Over the years, I had attended numerous programs and workshops on self-growth and spirituality. On this day, I was looking for some inspiration and renewal when the title The Seven Paths to the Soul caught my eye.

I called a friend who had already mentioned the workshop to me, and said that I wanted to go. I felt strangely compelled, as if

I had to go. But having made that decision, I felt, once again, the old conflict arise: there I was, once again, torn between addressing my needs and the needs of the rest of the family. The workshop lasted for ten days. As it turned out, the children were away at summer camp that week; it would have been a perfect week to spend some time with my partner, I thought regretfully. I was not in great shape, that is to say, I was in quite a bit of pain and very stiff. I was also going through many ups and downs physically and emotionally. I tried to persuade myself simply to stay home and rest, but somehow, the idea of the workshop had seized me; I could not let it go.

Instinctively, I felt that this workshop would be very important to me and I had to follow up its thread, its promise. I registered, and Chris drove me down to Tatamagouche. He carried my bag inside, and nearly carried me in as well. The friend who had encouraged me to do this workshop had already arrived. The setting was wonderful, beautiful and peaceful. We waited to see what would happen. The workshop was facilitated by three women: Olga Denisko, who was Director of Psychosynthesis Pathways in Montreal, Jean Hardy, a Psychosynthesis practitioner and the author of *A Psychology with a Soul: Psychosynthesis in Evolutionary Context*, who had come from England to do the workshop with Olga and with Rosemary Sullivan, another Psychosynthesis practitioner from Quebec, who worked primarily with incest survivors at a retreat center in the country.

As they soon explained, the concept of "seven paths to the soul" had its origins in Eastern spiritual traditions. Over the course of one's life, one might pursue several or all of the paths, because different moments in one's life sometimes required different avenues to spiritual growth. As we learned, the seven paths were Will, Action, Love, Beauty, Science, Ritual, and Devotion. The workshop was designed to give us the opportunity to explore these themes, and to see where and how they might fit in our lives. This workshop was my first introduction to Psychosynthesis and to Olga Denisko. Both were to become very important to me in coming days and years.

I was very impressed by Olga, recognizing in her an

enormously powerful, gifted teacher, healer and therapist. I was also very deeply struck by the psychosynthetic approach to psychology, in which human beings are not simply bundles of nerves and impulses, but souls who evolve towards ever greater wholeness. Psychosynthesis thus sought to draw one towards the richness and power of the higher unconscious; it offered a series of methods and techniques designed to help access the higher self.

Here again was another missing piece! I thought. All these years I had been striving towards something, but I did not quite know what to call it. As the workshop got underway, I was very excited for I had the sense that I had stumbled on to something very important. Although, I must say, "stumble" is not quite the right word. I was in that wonderful state of being in the right place at the right time—and there was no coincidence.

Despite my growing belief that I was meant to be there at this workshop, I had a very hard time being able to relax and to let myself be there. I had still not let go of my habits of restless activity and relentless second-guessing, of guilt and anxiety. I continued to feel turmoil over the decision I had made to go to the workshop. Oh, I should have stayed home and spent time with my partner, I thought. He had a week off and we could have had some quiet time together without the children. It was very hard, I found, to be with myself. I was still very angry, very much fighting the illness; I was desperately seeking a cure that would come from outside myself. I was utterly unaware that I had some inner work, and some personal healing to undertake, that I had to begin to work through some of the issues of abandonment that I carried with me since my childhood. The Seven Paths workshop was not only an introduction to Psychosynthesis for me but was also the beginning of that healing work that I had to do.

As we began our investigation of the seven paths, I soon realized that Will and Action had predominated in my life up to the point of my illness. Beauty and Ritual were also strong. I had some work to do to understand my use of these paths and their importance to me. I also had to consider that there might be some other routes as well involved in my spiritual evolution.

That week, the most powerful experience for me was some

imagery and journeying work that I did around the notion of Will. As I was eventually to discover, Will is a very important concept for Psychosynthesis. Assagioli wrote in detail about what he called the importance of "the act of will." Will, he wrote, was "the unknown and neglected factor in modern psychology, psychotherapy, and education," neglected, paradoxically, because of its very centrality to the conception of the self. In his work, he developed an analysis of the stages of the will, from intention, deliberation, decision, and affirmation of one's acts of will, to planning and what he called "direction of the execution of the will" or the capacity to combine both driving energy and persistence. On the basis of this analysis of the component parts of will, Assagioli elaborated techniques that would aid in the development and training of the will; the goal was to enable "the complete, effective, successful, volitional act, and use of the will, i.e., the total will in action." Over the course of my training, I came to recognize the distortions of my will, and the ways that those distortions led me into fruitless conflict with myself and others.

Those first exercises and the imagery work that we did on the Will provoked many insights for me. During the course of one exercise in guided visualization, a sort of heroine's journey, we were asked the question, "What do you long for most?" I answered, "Relationship, connection." To the question, "What is your purpose in life?" my answer was "Service to others." When asked to allow an image to emerge that represented our life's purpose for us, the image that came to me was the chalice or the Holy Grail. I was quite started by the emergence of this image from my unconscious; although it is a very archetypal Christian symbol, I also wanted to view it as another archetype, that of a female symbol, of the womb, the vessel of life. As I imagined it, the chalice was encrusted with jewels; at first I did not want to accept what seemed such extravagance; it seemed altogether too pretentious.

As it went on, the visualization experience took me though a process of recognizing what my purpose was, then losing sight of it. In the journeying I come up against many blocks and barriers as I made my way though a forest. I was told there would be a guide along the way who would give me tools to help me on my journey. The tools that I received included a sword, which I did not want at first because it seemed too masculine, and a gold ball set in a disk. The sword was to cut through illusion, and learning this, I was able to accept it, while the gold ball in the disk represented truth.

With these tools in hand, I forged my way though the forest until I reached a cave where a Darth Vader sort of figure blocked the entrance. He said to me, when I wanted to enter the cave, "You can't do this; you're not good enough," but then the light of clarity from my sword pushed him back, and I was able to gain entrance to the cave. I proceeded through the cave, and into a garden where adults and children played together in happiness and harmony. I found the grail in this garden, and although the richness of the jewels on it disturbed me, I mounted my horse with the sword, grail, ball and disk, and returned to my home. When I arrived, my family appeared to be overwhelmed by all that I brought with me. They turned their backs on me and walked away. But when they saw how happy I was, they soon returned.

This brief exercise in visualization spelled out for me the importance of the quest for the true self, the imperative to find the soul's path, and thus the purpose of the journey in this life. The visualization helped me to see that I might return with my purpose, the grail, a spiritual chalice, and that already I possessed some important tools: the sword that cuts through illusion and the ball and disk of truth. These were just what I needed—powerful tools for my journey.

A year or so later, in the fall of 1993, I enrolled in a foundation year program in Psychosynthesis. The year at massage school with all its changes, challenges, and hardships had propelled me into a new stage of spiritual growth, and I could not be content to stand still. The next three years of the training program in Psychosynthesis helped me to focus on what my life's work would be. It aided my understanding of the healing that I needed to do; it illuminated the limits of my survivor self and the distortions of my will; it brought me closer to the realization of my emerging path of love for myself and others. I had worked for many years with women in trauma in the Battered Women's

Shelter, I had wrestled with my own traumas, but until I undertook Psychosynthesis training, I knew that I didn't have the skills to do the deep work necessary to help myself or the women I had seen get on with their lives and grow and prosper. I was able to offer comfort, but I did not know anything about how to work with anger, split off parts of the personality, or dissociation. Psychosynthesis training encouraged me to face up to and make use of my emotions in my healing; it also taught me how to help others to do so as well.

As I pursued my training, it became clear to me how much I had been held back by my limited beliefs about myself. "The self is already attained," but so often we do not know it, and we turn away from our sources of strength, our wisdom, our soul's true path. We are preoccupied by other, apparently more immediate, things. Over the years of my training, I continued what had already been an extensive practice of reading about and exploring human potential and spiritual potential—the path of self-actualization that Maslow had so persuasively described in *Towards a Psychology of Being.*

Psychosynthesis with its focus on activating the higher unconscious and higher self was exactly the model of psychology I had been searching for. It made perfect sense, and echoed the beliefs of other influential wisdom traditions. Assagioli, its founder, believed, as many of these wisdom traditions also contended, that our basic nature is divine, that God or the spirit is within us; it is not other than we are. We are divine, and of the divine. As the Chandogya Upanishad holds:

> *In this very being of yours, you do not perceive the true, but there, in fact, it is. In that which is the subtle essence of your being, all that exists has its self. An invisible and subtle essence is the spirit of the whole universe. That is the **true**, that is the **self**, and **thou, thou art that**.*

The transcendence of the small self or survival self is the discovery of the big self or higher self, which is God. We all have moments in our lives where we glimpse this other reality, and seize a consciousness of higher selfhood, a moment where we step outside of our everyday worries and consciousness and enter the flow of the universe. This is what had happened to me in my room in Massachusetts that dark night when I passed from such deep despair to a blissful, transcendent state. It was a spontaneous occurrence, I could not reproduce it at will. But as I learned, in various of the Eastern traditions that so interested Assagioli, mystics, gurus, and rishis had developed practices that allowed one intentionally to open into such experiences, meditation, a calming of the self in order to listen deeply, being perhaps the most important among mystical techniques designed to access the higher consciousness or states of enlightenment. Meditation, contemplation, and prayer all call us into a state of stillness and inner connection. When we let go of our busy outer-directed focus and come to stillness, we are able to open at will to this other awareness within us that affirms our divine essence.

As Assagioli wrote of such "transpersonal" or spiritual states, in a passage that I've already mentioned:

> *Very often there is a sense of enlightenment, a new unearthly light which transfigures the external world and a light which reveals a new beauty. It illuminates the inner world, throws light on problems and doubts and dispels them. It is the intuitive light of a higher consciousness.*

In the process of my Psychosynthesis training, claiming my spiritual life and developing my spiritual self was the most empowering, inspiring, and healing experience of my life. God ceased to be some awful and repressive force outside of me; the divine, I learned, was within. We are and have always been that which we most long for. In us is the sacred and inherently good, and that goodness is the force of love which sustains the universe. As a Hasidic saying puts it,

> *A person is afraid of things that cannot harm us, and we know it. And we long for things that cannot help us and we*

know it. But actually, it is something within us that we are afraid of and it is something within us that we long for.

What wonderful, terrifying news!

LEARNINGS AND MEDITATIONS

THE SOUL'S PATH

Meditation on self: the center of pure consciousness and will.

Learnings
Meditations

In my experience of Psychosynthesis the most powerful learning tool was what Assiogili called the Self-Identification exercise. I learned that I had many parts, inside me, and at anytime I could be overwhelmed or over identified with any particular part. The sad wounded one, the rebel, and the survivor one. Anything we over identify with can control us. But we can learn to dis-identify (not disassociate) from any sub-personality or from any personality vehicle i.e. mind, body, feelings – and step back to the observer – center. The self – the I space which has a direct line to the divine. One of the most profoundly powerful learnings was to know I could step back and connect with this powerful centered space and in so doing direct and harmonize from the energy of this center.

Meditation on Self-Identification
The Observer centered I space

Seated comfortably bring your attention inside, connect with your breath, rest in your breathing. Become aware of a quiet space within you. Breathe and relax.

And now if you are willing, allow your self to become aware of your body – for some time just notice any body sensations in a natural way – just observe them and know that your body is a very precious instrument of experience in the world. It can hold sensations of great delight and utmost pain – it is a precious instrument of experience and action in the world, and say to yourself: <u>I am my Body and I am more than my Body</u>. Attempt to realize this as an experienced fact in your consciousness and let that go and <u>move</u> to the next step.

Now, allow yourself to be aware of your emotions – just notice any emotions present for you – and know that your emotions change – they ebb and flow from love to hatred from calm to anger – joy to sorrow – they may overwhelm you at times. But just observe them now and say, "<u>I have emotions and I am more than my emotions.</u>" Since I can observe my emotions I know they are not my self – I can learn to direct, utilize and integrate them harmoniously in my life and let that go and move to the next step.

Allow yourself to be aware of your mind – your streams of thought that come and go – the busy mind – the mind of knowledge, ideas, and experience. Be aware of this powerful <u>tool of discovery</u> and expression and know "<u>I have a mind and I am more than my mind</u>" and let that go and move to the next step.

*Having dis-identified with emotions, thoughts and sensations of the body – I ask myself who am **I**? I recognize and affirm that I am a center of pure consciousness and will. Attempt to realize this as an experienced fact in your awareness. And know you can use the energy of this center to direct and harmonize the content of mind, body and feelings. I am a center of pure consciousness and will.*

Breathe and rest.

CHAPTER VI

Grieving

When my illness first struck me, and for years afterward, there were days when I could not eat, and days when I could not speak. I cried endless tears, and withdrew from the world. What stands out most for me from the diary entries that I wrote at Stillpoint is the strength and persistence of the theme of abandonment and loss. That year, I began the work of re-experiencing my own pain and suffering as well as the pain and suffering of my mother and my sister. I felt at once both terrified—would I end up as they had?—and, strangely, freed. At last, I had begun to touch upon aspects of a pain that had been closed off for many many years, and I plunged into the most intense grieving. My sessions with the acupuncturist seemed to open these channels of sorrow. Astonished often, I found myself experiencing a profound sense of loss and grief, a sense which up to that time had been absent from my life.

As I have discussed, I had not been encouraged as a child to name any experience of sadness. It seemed that my mother would not tolerate it. She trained us to pull ourselves together, never to give in to emotion, always to battle on. *Grief, sadness*, and *loss* were not tolerated. The emotions that she had repressed and shut off in herself, she could not and would not allow in her children or those around her. Her anger and rage stayed with her all her life, and in the end consumed her.

As I have learned, anger and grief together form a two-headed beast. I myself had spent many years of my life wrestling with anger. My anger was not an everyday, all day, unable to enjoy life kind of anger, however, which is one of the ways that I lived with it. I guess I was angry a lot, but I was also aware that this anger had a force, that it was part of a necessary energy, fuel for the work of social change that I did. I had spent almost twenty years working as a feminist and in the peace movement. And every single one of the social justice issues that I fought for was outside of me; in all those years, I had not come to peace within. I could not, I think, come to peace with myself.

When I returned to Stillpoint from visiting my sister in England, my anger was renewed. Now it was about my illness, but it is also the case that I was discharging old anger and was deeply immersed in grief. All of these emotions poured from me in the course of my acupuncture sessions. Somehow I knew that this discharge was important, to feel these things at last was important, and so when I returned to Nova Scotia, I began a series of acupuncture sessions in Halifax. My acupuncturist told me that he would work with the lungs, which were associated with grief. In Massachusetts, my acupuncturist had been working with the earth and sympathy. I was not sure I was ready yet to work so closely with grief; I knew I could not control it. When I went for my sessions in Halifax, I walked into the acupuncturist's office—it would be more accurate to say that I hobbled in—and burst into tears. I was overwhelmed by my own outpouring of grief and sadness. I cried through entire sessions. I could barely walk. I could barely move. But twenty-five years after some of the most confusing events of my young life, I was learning how important it was to mourn my losses, including the loss of my emotionality, as well as the sensation of being abandoned in my terror and confusion.

What a healing balm at last being able to grieve was! I was

so open and vulnerable. My heart was unsealed. When I look back now, I realize that this massive outpouring of grief was the very beginning of the process in which I would be able to find peace within myself. It was an enormous step in my healing process. I had unleashed a dam; it was joined by the tributary waters of my current losses, which I also needed to grieve. All the physical activities that had given me so much pleasure—running, dancing, skiing—these were all in the past. The greatest loss was dancing, which I had loved to do with a passion.

Those first months after my diagnosis were a time of incredible emotional vulnerability. People around me had varying responses to my emotionality. In the Quaker group which I met with for silent prayer every second Sunday, I felt that I could share the depths of this gift that had come into my life. I gradually realized that the process I was going through was, however difficult, a wonderful gift of the universe; it was bringing me to a deeper level of awareness, to an opening of compassion. The opening of my heart allowed me to see that the essential message, a message that has been echoed through many spiritual traditions, was to open oneself to love. The call to be a lover in the universe is a call to see the profound wisdom and order and rightness of everything. Thus when we cease to struggle against change, our suffering diminishes. We are able to see that all is one.

Of course, at first, all of this was very difficult for me to deal with or to grasp. I remember, three years after the onset of my illness, going into the office of my acupuncturist in Halifax, who was a Buddhist. I said something to him about "when I was normal" again. He looked at me curiously and said, "Are you still caught up with what you were like when you were 'normal'? How long have you had arthritis?" When I replied, "Three years," he shook his head in gentle admonishment and reminded me that if I continued to live in the past and to struggle against change, that my suffering would increase rather than diminish.

But it was hard to heed such wisdom; I struggled with and against it for months and years. As long as I was intent on finding a cure and returning to my old 'healthy' self, I was not living in the present. And indeed, I wanted to get away from the present and this hideous thing that was happening to me. But because I was fleeing where I was, I could find no peace.

The enormous outpouring of grief that I began to experience in acupuncture sessions was the beginning of an acceptance of the way things were. And later, when I did Psychosynthesis training, I came to understand, even more, how to come into my body, how to be in my body and to stay grounded in the present. Alongside my training, I was reading widely about differing spiritual traditions. I was particularly drawn to the teachings of Buddhism through the writings of Pema Chödrön, a North American Buddhist nun, and the director of Gampo Abbey in Cape Breton, Nova Scotia. Her book *Start Where You Are* focussed on what she called "compassionate living" or learning to live in the present moment with whatever feelings are present within you. Pema contended that compassion starts with ourselves. She suggested avenues towards self-acceptance, avenues and spiritual exercises that helped me to accept and understand my anger, my jealousy, even my small-mindedness. Her words reminded me that the first step was to be gentle with myself, that I must start with self-acceptance—an acceptance of who I am at this very moment now, without making comparisons between myself and anyone else. Without wishing to be a better person. Without comparing myself with how I had been in the past or projecting into the future. Just accepting now.

Likewise, in my training as a Psychosynthesis psychotherapist, I was learning how important it was to be in the body, to be present in the emotion, and to stay with the pain, the fear, the anger that one felt. I was learning that it was essential not to suppress these unwanted aspects, but to befriend them. Thus, as I learned how to work with clients, I also undertook profound healing work with myself. I realized that living compassionately meant embracing the knowledge that all is one, that there is no separation between the terrible and lovely parts of ourselves, that they are all forms, more or less distorted, of ourselves. With this knowing comes the experience of wholeness and healing.

Today, when I work with clients who were traumatized as children, often a very important part of their work is to grieve the pain and loss of a childhood they never had, or of feelings and emotions they split off from. As was my experience, beneath the anger they have carried lies deep sadness and grief. Often enough, a person is even aware of this sadness in the guise of depression. Frequently, they have for many years been unable to break through the depression to the original feelings that they suppressed at a far earlier age. Working with clients on grief and anger means opening the door to re-experiencing these feelings and grieving their losses.

So many of us must go through the process that is very well documented in Alice Miller's book, *The Drama of the Gifted Child*. There, she describes depression as a defence against feeling emotions, and outlines how we create *false selves* that allow us to carry on and survive, but which deny or repress our true selves. We cover over our feelings of being wounded, we split off from such a sense of ourselves as "the wounded one." In fact, we may come to despise this part of our selves—as I did—the victim or child part that is weak and fearful, insecure and vulnerable.

It was this part of me that cried for days, that could not speak, that withdrew from the world. But finally, I realized that I had a right to experience these feelings as fully as I wished, that my feelings were not dysfunctional, but suppressing them was. I need not feel weak and inadequate because I had these emotions. I need not feel I have to overcome them; in fact I could embrace them and in so doing, free myself.

In this way, along the path of lived experience, came my understanding of the profound importance of the grieving process to any healing journey. It was with great relief that I realized I would never have to suppress this part of my emotional life again; I promised myself that I would value and honour these feelings as much as my feelings of joy, peace, or contentment. I would not run away from so-called "negative emotions" anymore.

LEARNINGS AND MEDITATIONS

GRIEF – The Heart of Sadness

Learnings
Meditations

In the human journey fear, loss and grieving are common to us all. With any change comes loss and we experience the pain in our heart. In allowing grief to enter our lives we allow the movement forward of healing. Many of us may experience a withholding – resentment and anger at the injustice of it all. On a personal and a global level there is much loss to mourn but when we allow our pain we move forward on our journey to freedom. We surrender our sadness to the heart of light.

Heart of Light Meditation

Seated comfortably bring your attention inside. Connect with your breath – rest in your breathing. Become aware of a quiet space within. Notice your body and bring your attention to your heart area – that space between the breasts where you sense a pressure or heaviness. Notice this heaviness which seems to be blocking the spaciousness beneath. You may notice an ache that carries the losses and fears of a lifetime. Allow yourself to feel it – open to it. Place your hand gently on this place. Feel the pain in your heart, breathe into it. Allow yourself to go deeper – feel the sufferings you hold there. Continue to hold your hand over this spot, notice any resistance or armoring. Allow the resistance to soften and melt open to the deepest grief, feel the isolation or abandonment, the lack of control over illness, death, loss of a loved one, fears of the unknown. Connect if you will with a loss, which is particularly poignant right now. Let yourself experience it – just as it is. Let go into the pain, bring it into awareness of the compassionate heart. Beneath it – the courage and compassion that it is always there. Feel the heart expanding. The pain just floating there. Allow the soft heart energy to surround the pain – softening and transforming it. Allow yourself to gently exhale – discharging the pain. Let it float away into the universe where it can transform and dissipate. Continue breathing into the newly awakened heart space – feel the sense of light and love – know your connection to the courage and compassion which is always within your heart.

Breathe and rest.

CHAPTER VII

Will: The Energy of Choice

I have written in some detail about my longing and my
search for the Divine within—my own quest for the Holy Grail.
And as I discussed in the last chapter, my deepest lesson in these
eleven years has been the importance of opening myself to and for
compassion. The softening and opening of my heart, the powerful
flood of unconditional love I experienced in my room in Massachusetts on that fateful night in my darkest hour, these were all
steps on my journey. Finally, at last, in this new awakening of
compassion and love, I could include myself. Loving and accepting myself in such a gentle friendly fashion was new for me, and it
did not come easily at first.

My strength of will had propelled me forward for many
years. My ability to focus my will to survive difficult situations
had been a very valuable asset; my ability to focus my will for
social action and justice work had been a big part of my life and
the lives of others. This work was fuelled by my anger and a deep
rage associated with my childhood, together with a desire to overcome the injustice I saw around me in the world.

Despite its force and strength, however, my will was distorted because it was focussed primarily on power and control. Never again would I allow myself to be controlled by another. In turn, I would wield power and be in control. In many areas of my life I was stubborn, inflexible, and intolerant. I had to be in control in personal relationships—of course this is where my inflexibility caused the most difficulty. In those days of my strength of will, what I had yet to learn was compassion for myself—that I could soften and embrace those hurt parts of me that needed to be in control, and that I could acknowledge the fear that lay beneath the hurt. What did the hurt part of me need in order to allay its fears of abandonment and annihilation? Getting at and then answering such questions were a part of what in Psychosynthesis is called the "subpersonality" work, work on the different aspects of our many "selves" that I did in my therapy. As I went through the three-year training we worked through the steps of awareness, acknowledge-ment, re-parenting, re-framing, and integrating these fractured aspects of myself toward a unity or synthesis.

As I got more in touch with the whole of my self, my higher self and my divine nature, I began to realize I would never be alone. Once I had developed an awareness of the larger spiritual or transpersonal aspect of myself, once I knew that I was one with the ALL, how could I be abandoned, how could I be alone?

Naturally this development was difficult—and is, even now. It is hard to give up years of living out fearful patterns, to face one's fears and overcome them. But the more that I realized the power of the spirit manifested in my open heart, the easier it was for me to embrace the knowledge of my own basic goodness. And once I could do that, I was more and more able to let go of fear and the anger it produced. I came to feel that I was okay, that to be was enough. I could relax and be more God/ess-centered; this was a viable and important activity for life. Slowly, as I worked, I struggled to realize, in the deepest part of me, that I am whole, loving, and loveable.

Such a renewed understanding of self, will, and the divine enables me to be more compassionate with myself, and it opens me still further to compassionate action in the world, and in service to others, which also increases my understanding of good will and compassionate action. The whole acts like a wonderful and perfect feedback loop.

When I write, I struggle with activating my will. Or when I am recovering from surgery, I need my will to push myself to do rehabilitation exercises, to push through the pain. As I struggle with my will before the page, I convince myself to write about what I have learned, what it means, why it is important. I persuade myself to write it now, today. Just get it down. Another day I will re-organize it, edit it so that it makes sense and flows in sequence.

These are the challenges that face the skilful will. Working by skilful means, one saves time and effort. The qualities inherent in the skilful will are endurance, mastery and discipline, organization, and integration. Planning, organizing, and disciplining myself to do this writing means using skilful will "to develop that strategy which is most effective and which entails the greatest economy of effort" (Assagioli, 1992).

In learning more about the power of Will, I have become aware that I can *choose* how to respond to any given situation in my life. I know that I do not have to be a victim of circumstance without any say in how I respond or how I make meaning out of my experience. Every day I make choices, and my life is the result of making many choices over time.

Sometimes, admittedly, these choices are made unconsciously, or consciously but not carefully or truthfully, as in times when I am convinced by the feelings of others around me or by the expectations of family and friends to do something that it is not really in my heart to do. Or when I succumb to pressures to think and be a certain way that fits the status quo, rather than having the courage to seek my own direction. Those times when I have *consciously* and carefully made difficult decisions that went against others' expectations, but which were true and right for me, have been powerful, affirming experiences. In such moments, I have felt that my choice emanated from the deepest center of myself. And as Assagioli has argued, "where the will is, there also is one's center, one's self." (Assagioli, 1992)

Positive attributes of a strong will lead to actions that are determined, courageous, decisive, persistent, the meaningful and directed pursuit of one's goals. A distortion of strong will is manifest when someone behaves in inflexible ways, when I am (as I so often have been and often still am) stubborn, headstrong, unbending and obstinate. As Assagioli so wisely described it,

> *The most effective and satisfactory role of the will is not as a source of direct power and force but as a function which can stimulate, regulate and direct all other functions and forces of our being so that they may lead us to our predetermined goal.* (Assagioli, 1992)

When we work with clients and when we do our own healing work, utilizing the will is an integral part of making choices for change. As Alice Miller so poignantly describes in her book *For Your Own Good*, breaking the child's will—before she is even aware that she has a will—has been the focus of a good number of destructive pedagogical and child-raising practices. As Miller says, such "practices are still present to some degree today in the guise of 'disciplining' the child."

In our work, clients may talk about the effects of trauma or abuse in their childhoods, events that crippled their will. Learning about different aspects of will, and practicing activity of will is thus an important part of their healing work. The first step in recovering, or developing, a skilful will is awareness of one's patterns of behaviour. What blocks you, what holds you back? In addition to individual therapy, I now also offer my clients a spiritual growth study group. In this group setting I present information and exercises on working with the Will; we learn about dis-identification, self-identification, and other important aspects of Psychosynthesis theory and practice. We also use meditation as a tool for grounding and spiritual practice.

Because it is a study group, we cultivate an atmosphere that is curious, open, and flexible. It is possible in such a setting to bring in readings from many sources to develop and elaborate on any specific topic or theme. In the course of our work, I have learned something that I also seek to teach: above all, Psychosynthesis is an empowerment model of psychotherapy. It identifies and celebrates the natural tendency of our nature to move toward wholeness; it is not grounded in pathology.

If we know how we may look, everywhere in the world around us we see movement toward wholeness or greater synthesis. There is an implicit order that propels everything in nature: to restore, re-dress, and renew itself. From the simple example of how a cut finger heals itself, we may move to wonder at this complex, spiritually rich, and miraculous process of life, which as yet we do not fully understand. Transpersonal psychology brings us back, not simply to mundane reality, but to our divine essence.

In our study group we explore those aspects of ourselves that unite us to all beings of all times. We strive to become familiar with the universal themes that all beings struggle with: pain, suffering, anger, attachment, illness, death, impermanence, separation, love, beauty, joy, creativity.

We pass into mystical states from out of ordinary consciousness, as from less into more, as from smallness into vastness, and at the same time from unrest to rest. We feel them as reconciling unifying states. They appeal to the yes function more than the no function in us.

We allow the creative force of the universe to develop and deepen, and we honour this creative force within ourselves. In this way, we may grow and thrive; we cultivate and sow greater understanding and joy. It is not despite suffering, but thanks to it sometimes, that we are brought into greater wholeness and light. As the Mundaka Upanishad suggests:

Self is everywhere, shining forth from all beings, vaster than the vast, subtler than the most subtle, unreachable yet nearer than breath, than heartbeat. Eye cannot see it, ear cannot hear it, nor tongue utter it. Only in deep absorption can the mind, grown pure and silent, merge with the formless truth. As soon as you find it, you are free, you have found yourself. You have solved the great riddle. Your heart forever is at peace. Whole, you enter the whole. Your personal self returns to its radiant intimate deathless source.

LEARNINGS AND MEDITATIONS

FREEDOM TO CHOOSE – *Living Willingly*

Learnings
Meditations

"How often before we begin have we declared a task impossible? How often have we believed ourselves inadequate? A great deal depends upon the thought patterns we choose and the persistence with which we affirm them." These are the words of Piero Ferucci, student of Assagioli, from his book "What We May Be". He is referring to the use of will – living <u>willingly</u>, conscious effort and <u>conscious choice</u>. Which thought patterns do you affirm in your life? In what ways do you hold yourself back? I can't change… I can't try that; this job is too difficult for me, etc…. We discover and activate our will by <u>using</u> it in the simplest ways in our everyday lives. What changes do you want to make? Don't be afraid to reach for your dreams – with determined effort and will anything is possible.

Meditation on Willing

Take a moment now to relax and go inside – connect with your *breath. Rest in your breathing, become aware of a quiet space within. Take a moment to connect with and become aware of a situation in your life in which you wish to make a change. See yourself in that situation – and connect now with your center, your deepest self – your deepest, quietest place. Feel the energy and power of that center. See yourself hold the posture and dignity of "willing" to make the change you need to make. Feel the presence of the power of will in your mind, body and feelings and say to yourself: <u>I am; I can; I will.</u> Repeat this as you see yourself making the change you wish to make. See yourself completing the tasks using skilful means for the support of your highest good and the good of others. See yourself successfully completing the steps of making change or getting the project done. Feel the power of this focused determination, this conscious choice to achieve your goal. Feel and know the joy of completing this task. Feel the joy that is the highest quality of the will.*

Breathe and rest.

Use this meditation to prepare for any act of will. Practice acts of will daily. Open to the realms of possibility.

Breathe and rest.

EPILOGUE

There are many stories in any one person's life time and there is always fear to overcome in putting this often very private information out in the world. When we speak about what really matters we get close to matters of the heart—Joy, Sorrow, Love, Beauty, Fear, Pain—all these potent life experiences.

At this point I feel a deep sense of gratitude for all that life has given to me. The many challenges have brought me closer to myself and to others. My heart knows no bounds. I remember reading somewhere that the most important task we must learn in any lifetime is to open to love. To love as deeply, simply, fearlessly as we can. Of course we may have heard this many times and wondered why it is so hard to do. Mostly because our fears, vulnerability, small-mindedness and at the deepest level our feelings "I am not enough" hold us back. I am not good enough. Lies, all lies. We must begin now to celebrate ourselves (the other great task of a life time) with gentle loving kindness. We must *be* the love we wish to see in the world.

My wish for you, dear reader, is that you grow in love, beauty and awareness of your true nature, your basic goodness. My best wishes, love and salutations to you on your journey.

N'ameste... Barbara Hayes *September 2001*

BIBLIOGRAPHY/SUGGESTED READINGS

Assagioli, R.   *The Act Of Will*, Arkana: Penguin, 1992.

Assagioli, R.   *Psychosynthesis A Manual Of Principles and Techniques*, New York: Penguin, 1965.

Assagioli, R.   *Transpersonal Development: The Dimension Beyond Psychosynthesis*, Harper/Collins, 1993.

Chödrön, P.   *Start Where You Are: A Guide to Compassionate Living*, Boston: Shambhala, 1994.

Dossey, L.   *Healing Words: The Power Of Prayer and The Practice Of Medicine*, New York: Harper/Collins, 1993.

Duff, K.   *The Alchemy of Illness*, New York: Bell Tower (Crown Books), 1993.

Ferrucci, Piero.   *What We May Be: Techniques for Psychological and Spiritual Growth Through Psychosynthesis.* Jeremy P. Tarcher Inc. Los Angeles, 1982.

Frankl, V.   *Man's Search for Meaning*, Boston: Beacon Press, 1963.

Grof, S.   *Realms Of The Human Unconscious: Observed From L.S.D. Research*, New York: E.P. Dutton, 1976.

Hardy, J.   *A Psychology With a Soul: Psychosynthesis in Evolutionary Context*, London: Woodgrange, 1996.

Huxley, A.   *Doors Of Perception*, New York: Harper, 1990.

James, W.   *The Varieties Of Religious Experiences*, New York: The Modern Library, 1929.

Maslow, A.   *Toward A Psychology Of Being*, Van Nostrand, 1968.

Miller, A.   *The Drama of the Gifted Child: The Search for the True Self*, New York: HarperCollins, 1994.

Miller, A.   *For Your Own Good: Hidden Cruelty In Child Rearing and the Roots Of Violence*, New York: Noonday Press, 1990.

Remen, R.N.   *Kitchen Table Wisdom: Stories that Heal*, New York: Riverhead Books, 1996.

Rilke, R.M.   *Letters To A Young Poet*, NewYork: W.W. Norton & Co., 1993.

Ring, K.   *Heading Toward Omega: In Search Of The Meaning Of Near Death Experience*, New York: William Morrow, 1984.

Siegel, B.   *Love, Medicine and Miracles: Lessons Learned about Self-healing from a Surgeon's Experience with Exceptional Patients*, New York: Harper and Row, 1986.

Starhawk,   *Dreaming The Dark: Magic Sex and Politics*, Boston: Beacon Press, 1982.

Stone, M.   *When God Was a Woman*, New York: Harcourt, Brace, Jovanovich, 1976.

Upanishad, Chandogya.

Upanishad, Mundaka.

Whitman, W.   *The Complete Poems*, New York: Penguin, 1975.

Wilber, K. and Treya Killam Wilber, *Grace And Grit*, Boston: Shambhala, 1990.

* M. Williamson, quoted by Nelson Mandela. Cited by Jean Hardy in *A Psychology with a Soul: Psychosynthesis in Evolutionary Context*, epigraph.